From A

Zen

Uncovering the Core of My Anxiety and Reclaiming My Life

Marilyn Mendoza

chipmunkapublishing
the mental health publisher

Published by
Chipmunkapublishing
PO Box 6872
Brentwood
Essex CM13 1ZT
United Kingdom

http://www.chipmunkapublishing.com

Edited by Kirsty Burlton

Chipmunkapublishing gratefully acknowledge the support of Arts Council England.

Acknowledgements

The author gratefully acknowledges quotes used in the chapter "Master Class"
"From the book The four Agreements" © 1997, Miguel Angel Ruiz, M.D. Reprinted by permission of Amber-Allen Publishing, Inc. P.O Box 6657, San Rafael CA.94903. All rights reserved."

The author also wishes to thank www.nyc-architecture and www.esential-architecture.com for the image of the Williamsburg Housing Project

For my children, Elena, Jason, Jonas, Junette-Desiree and my loving partner Jackson for their love and understanding.

I also want to thank Nanise Young for her positive and unwavering support and encouragement for my memoir and her excellent proofreading help

Finally, my book is dedicated to my mother Edith Chalfin Mendoza whose love for me was stronger than her illness

Prologue

Angie is missing. He didn't call. Carl is very worried. Carl is so worried about both of us. He said he wished he were dead. Between the two of us, I never should have come home from the hospital. He never should have taken in Angie. He meant well. His life is coming apart. I wonder where Angie is. He was very sick when he left. Carl doesn't know what to do. If I were well I would. It is not even 6 o'clock. I called Sally and upset her. Ray called and for the first time I told her I was very sick. It is 6 o'clock. I am very sick. It is only 6 o clock? No pills till 9. I don't know what to do. I don't feel like writing tonight. I always hated to write... Why did the doctor tell me to write a journal? Goodnight and God help all of us, Amen.

PART 1

THE WAY OUT IS THROUGH THE DOOR YOU CAME IN

R.D LAING
SCOTTISH PSYCHIATRIST 1927-1989

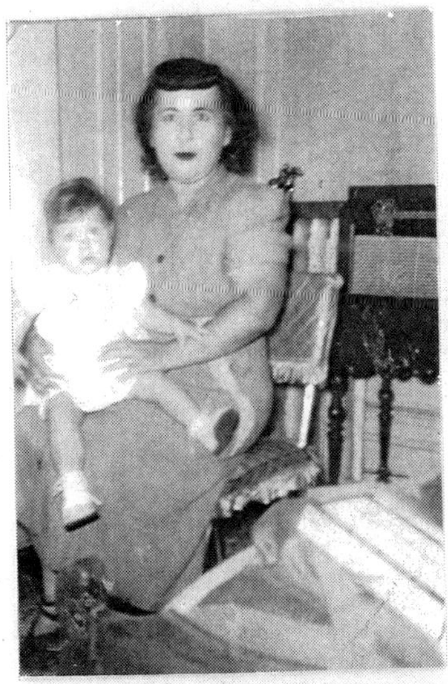

CHAPTER 1

YOU CAN'T COVER THE SKY WITH YOUR HAND (NO SE PUEDE TAPAR EL CIELO CON LA MANO) -- A PUERTO RICAN SAYING

It was August 24, 1970, my nineteenth birthday, a year after the summer of love ended with a fatality at the Rolling Stones free Altamont California concert, and I was about to be raped and murdered.

"Everyone likes you in the beginning, but when they get to know you, they want to smash in your smiley face." I stopped and stared for a minute. Had the fool actually said something meaningful? I was so giddy to be rid of my husband Jose that I carried his suitcase six blocks to the 18th Avenue train station in Bensonhurst, Brooklyn.

Before this I was barely listening. "You know I love you; why'd you make me hurt you." Blah, Blah, Blah. He was referring to the last Saturday when I gave him a jar filled with my home made potato salad for dinner. I was partying in Central Park with my friends, picking up my daughter at my mother's afterwards. He ate the damn thing before tossing the empty jar at me with such force it barely missed Elena in her baby carriage. How dare I not serve him a proper meal at the table and in a jar yet? And where was I all day, with Frenchie? He had stolen my diary during our last breakup and read, "The business with Frenchie is over." Was I still seeing Frenchie? I didn't respond until he said…

"All you care about is reading and eating."

"All you care about is pot and standing on the corner, rain or shine with your worthless friends."

His disregard for our daughter Elena was the catalyst that drove me to kick him out this time; not the ten black stitches sewed into the gaping wound in my thigh. He called the ambulance against my protests when we couldn't stop the bleeding. They didn't believe my story that it was an accident. I kept the secret but we knew he had to leave, so here I was listening to his whiny voice and carrying the rocks he seemed to be bringing out of my house. I tried to forget him and instead concentrate on the fun I would have when he left with his smelly socks and beer breath. It was almost worth the scars to be free again.

That night we were going to a new place for me, "The Village Gate" the legendary jazz cavern which tonight featured Latin jazz.

As we took the F train, facing us was a threesome of undetermined sex, age or species. I only peeked at the one with a charred face and red fright wig. Too afraid of directly looking at them, out of my peripheral vision, I noticed they were pointing and laughing at us. The thought would have been amusing if I wasn't about to pee my pants.

Then one said, "The one with the nose is Barbara Streisand and the blonde with all the makeup looks like Bridget Bardot's ugly sister."

I felt a bad omen knock out some of the boundless air in my balloon but thankfully they got off at the stop before West Fourth Street.

My mood changed the moment the night air hit me. I was pretty again and the air breathed sweetness on my skin. I was wearing hip hugger vertically striped Chic jeans which I paired with my own invention, a tight purple vest-sans blouse crushing my breasts and revealing bare skin. I was being called out by girls and boys alike with, "Hey I like your top, nice."

"Thanks man," I was taught always to be polite.

I had thought of this nude look to showcase my flat stomach. It had been a year since giving birth to my first child and gaining forty pounds. I lost it with the popular

Stillman diet, basically meat and an ocean of water and although I had lost my concave stomach, the 70's equivalent of a six pack, I celebrated my new body and birthday at a boutique when I reached 115 pounds. Tonight would be my debut.

The focal point of my ensemble wasn't the top or the pants. It was my "Lady Aerosmith" shoes which set me back a hundred bucks -worth every penny. I shopped at the Manhattan store, where I always seemed to be the only blonde among glamorous caramel and ebony skinned women. I crept in shyly and slithered out feeling bold and well, tall. Tonight, I towered over five foot three Linda, in my masterpiece of confidence. These beauties were constructed of what surely must have been steel; the two inch foundation and entire base shone like black diamonds and were topped with hand painted glitter and stars in red, white and blue. I was more patriotic then.

I was magic that night, held up in six inches of power, and didn't need my usual ruse of covering my acne with my hair. I let it flow free, and floated my curvy ass down that street. My only fear; that no one would ask me to dance; being a "wall flower" as my mother called it always lurked in the back of my mind.

Every Friday night placed most of our crowd at the "Corso" on East 86th street and Third Avenue, in Manhattan, where the bands were loud and well known and more importantly, the guys outnumbered the girls. Linda, Cassandra, Rosa and Ana would first gather at my house after my favorite sitcom, "That girl" with Marlo Thomas. Before they arrived, I watched the BBC Granada television show "A Family at War" and imagined I was Sheila; unhappily married and in bed with a RAF fighter pilot.

Then Cassandra would say, "Let's put Linda's make up on." So we all squeezed into my tiny bathroom fighting for my one small mirror, among a haze of Chanel No.5 and sweet sweat. One of us stayed behind, and turned up the 8 -Track tape so we could hear the Salsa music blasting across my apartment. Linda finally emerged looking surprised at the amount of makeup Puerto Rican girls can pile on. I usually let her use my stuff, because Linda never bought anything that could be gotten free. Afterwards it was time to practice our dancing. We squealed as we raced each other back to the living room.

I never learned how to put on false eyelashes; my emphasis was always hiding my acne scars. I used Helena Rubenstein foundation, carefully putting on enough to look more luminous than ghostly, not always succeeding. Then I put on my liquid eyeliner, no smudging allowed then. After that I carefully added wings to the end of my lids looking more like a fallen angel than a cat. Mascara and frosted pink lipstick completed my mask. My friends with perfect skin never used foundation. Rosa, the sex fiend in our group couldn't even pronounce it saying, "Marilyn did you put on your "consummation" yet? My friends all cracked up except me, knowing Rosa's caramel skin was pore-less. Hell, I thought, it will be dark in the club.

We left the house at 11:45 p.m. taking the train to Manhattan. Sometimes we would stop for a wine cooler at a nearby bar, making sure the club would be crowded when we made our entrance. We stood by the pole next to the live band which announced to the guys we were there to dance.

We once saw a group of ladies in their late twenties at a table nearby with a bottle of Bacardi and promised ourselves we would never be caught dead that old in a club let alone sitting down. We danced all night and never took the train home before the sun came up. I never drank the rum and Coke that was de rigueur at those venues or even stopped for water branding me a "camel" by my friends. My high was dancing with good smelling Latin men hoping for that illusive dancer who would make other dancers stop in their tracks on the floor to cheer us on. Rosa's high was men and booze and we all knew that although we left with her, she would never be on the train on the way back. She never considered it a good night unless she got laid. I once observed her dancing in a dark club with her Maxi coat opened to just panties and she later confessed she was screwing a guy on the dance floor. Those weren't the moves I hungered for. I loved the men twirling me around, feeling the heat of the music burn my soul.

Linda was my only Jewish friend and I met her through Cassandra Ramos, a project girl I had known since childhood. But it wasn't our mutual race that brought us together; it was our love of the Latin nightlife, the compulsion to dance to live Salsa bands. Salsa means sauce in Spanish, and Salsa music is a fusion of big band, Spanish, and African beats. In the 1970's, El Gran Combo of Puerto Rico and the original El Cantanete-Hector Lavoe, singer for Willie Colon, were the bands that turned us on. If I got lucky I sometimes scored a dance with a major player. I once danced with Larry Harlow and an Albino looking Latin singer, Nestor Sanchez who was in Tony Pabon Y La Protesta's band.

Tonight, Linda's mildly retarded sister Lainie babysat my daughter. I only used her when I was desperate. My mother always wanted to take Elena but she lived too far and I didn't need her putdowns before an evening out.

Linda wasn't conventionally pretty, but her looks were never the point. She had a well scrubbed face and a naturally slim figure and when she borrowed my clothes, she got dances. Her frizzy mane was acceptable when not nesting a family of lice she once presented to me. Her nose, a baby bird's beak fit her narrow face but the tip moved unpleasantly on its own when she spoke. Her claim to infamy was her strange laugh. She would break out in hyena-like guffaws at the most lame jokes. Our crowd kept her on as court jester, but because I was a stay at home mom and she had free access to a phone and freedom to lounge at her civil service job, we talked every day and had arrived at a place where I thought we were close.

Linda's parents threw her out of their house because of her preference for black men and partying. I had taken her in because that's what I do. She moved in with me and my baby daughter. I had a five room apartment in Bensonhurst, a step up and a long train ride from my first neighborhood, Williamsburg and my mother. I had planned this move and counted checks in an office in Manhattan for six months to earn the bribe of one thousand dollars the leaving tenants were demanding. To accomplish this, Jose and I moved in with my parents. When I came home from work I picked up Elena from her crib, and put on Janis Joplin's album, ok, maybe I did put on the album first.

Ma screamed at me, "You're a lousy mother and a worthless daughter," but I drowned her out with Janis' soulful rendition of "Ball and Chain", and "Down on Me." I was offered a raise after the three months of probation were up and quit the same day with a thousand dollars in my hand and the satisfaction of seeing my supervisor's surprised face.

My only goal was my mother's taunt-to live above my station in life.

I was free, young and invincible. Linda was cheap, naïve and a world traveler. She managed to save most of her paychecks and went on organized tours to different destinations every year. Her last trip had been to India and she paid four thousand dollars for that trip, a fortune to us at the time, hell at any time. She worked as a bookkeeper for the City, saving most of her paycheck and studied accounting at night at Brooklyn College. But the weekends belonged to us.

I had never been to the Village Gate though it was famous. In fact I rarely frequented the Village. I felt out of place with hippies and love, free or otherwise, and with anyone who couldn't understand my passion for red dresses and perfume.

Latin men would look at me with shocked faces when I declined their favorite line. "Do you want to smoke Yerba (pot) downstairs? "Yerba" never did it for me either. Nothing did, not getting married or even having a child the year before had given me the high dancing did.

That night we went to see Cal Tjader with Eddie Palmieri. When we entered "The Gate", the vibe was different from our usual places. There were groups of older people waiting for the jazz to start. I smelled a hint of uncertainty in the air. The diverse crowd was dressed in the best polyester Saks Fifth Avenue offered and my mood changed from confident to the familiar darkness that came with feeling not good enough. I draped my hair over my eyes, until the band started playing and the first dance offer came my way.

"We don't go home with anyone," I reminded Linda. We had a pact; that we stayed together no matter what. New York City was a dangerous place and I had been stranded too many times by girlfriends, usually Rosa, who hooked up with one night stands. Looking for deserted train stations in unfamiliar neighborhoods was getting old. Underneath, Linda's facade of respectability and humor lurked a dangerous innocence. She would bring guys back to my apartment and too many mornings my daughter would wake up to a stranger cooing at her. I accepted this behavior because that's also what I did.

We were dancing with two self proclaimed cousins and I had bad vibes about my dance partner. He was a small man of about twenty five with light caramel skin and few words. His quiet demeanor and mispronunciation of my fake Spanish name did not endear me to him since he said he was Puerto Rican. His fake name was Carlos. My fake name that night was Desiree. Tonight, Linda's fake name was Solly.
She would go into hysterics when she said, "I'm Solly, and this is Maria?" Not noticing that the guys didn't care what our names were. But it was fun to pretend to be someone else

"You look like a model," Carlos whispered in my ear.

"It's dark, I joked." Linda's conquest that night was the cousin, a cute black man with even white teeth over a jolly smile. He claimed to be a Soul Train dancer and that was huge to us, because every Saturday morning found us glued to the TV watching the famous "Soul Train dance line." At the end of the night, Linda captured me in a corner to plead her case.

"They want to drive us home." I didn't drink alcohol but the saxophones and trombones competed for my attention and the undercurrents of danger were blurred. I felt her hot breath on my face as she leaned in and shouted "please."
"No," I said automatically, "You know the rules." Her voice got whiny and even louder.

"These guys are so nice and we could save on train fare." It was all about saving money with her but money was not a draw for me so she pulled out her ace card, "We won't have to walk home from the train station and almost get mugged like the last time." In the din of the music I lost my reason and walked off to my destiny.

I felt a cloud slide over me like a death comforter the moment I entered the car. Linda was oblivious as usual. When we drove through dark streets and alleys to the river, I tried to calm myself but I lived in Brooklyn, and we weren't entering any freeway or street that looked familiar. We stopped as if by design and Linda and her new friend said they would take a walk along the river so I was stuck in the car alone with "Carlos".

"I just got discharged from the military-Turkey, dirty place, dirty women, wouldn't even look at me. All women are dirty and it was some dirty girl that got me dishonorably discharged when she accused me of stalking and threatening her," he said.

He took out what looked like a hunting knife and starting playing with it." This is my lucky knife - killed a few people with it."

He leaned in for a moment and I breathed in his essence.

"They deserved it -believe me." He spoke half to himself as he proceeded to arrange me on the seat in as prone a position as the Pinto car seat would allow. He held the knife in back of him, always hidden from my view but I felt it pressing against the back of my neck.

"Take off your pants," he said quietly. I obeyed- slipping wide bell bottom legs over the huge shoes and folding the pants carefully on the seat. He touched my panties. When I flinched he said, "What's wrong. What's wrong?"...

"Nothing."

Open your legs," he barked, and then I realized I had an immediate predicament added to my troubles. I had "hysterical vaginismus" which means the PC muscles in my vagina contracted automatically and I had never had sex with a man between my legs or ever had an internal examination, before, after or even giving birth. The obstetrician had to shine a big light to see the baby's head coming out.

Before I could think, he put one of my legs on the dashboard of the Pinto. I bent the other leg behind me praying my condition would not get me killed sooner. While his mouth pressed against mine I opened my mouth which was supposed to open my vaginal muscles.

"You're a sexy tight whore, you like it don't you?"

I nodded and felt the blade nick the back of my neck. I was silent and didn't plead with him, somehow knowing he would kill me if I did.

Then I tried to think of how I could live, knowing my survival depended on how I handled this time bomb, but my mind was frozen; what should I do next? I didn't want to die and leave my baby, my life, but how could I get through this?

In a dream like sequence, I remembered my mother telling my father that she would never commit suicide because she was Jewish. My father had been leaving for his usual weekend out and she was depressed. She told me that she was taught by her father that in Judaism the value of human life comes above almost any other commandment and she would never take her life.

Then, I heard her voice clear as a bell. "Live, Marilyn, no matter what, think and live."

He used the knife as silent persuasion. I wanted to scream and cry, but a clear knowledge that I needed to do something else to live invaded my consciousness. His breathing was heavy against my open mouth and I felt his irritation heighten when he couldn't enter me easily. Although I gave it a final painful try, my screaming muscles protested the indignity and I couldn't spread my legs to his satisfaction.

"Open wider," he sounded angry now, so I tried again. The fake leather was cold against my body. He finally collapsed on top of me with a shout, pulling my hair, the side of the knife pressing my throat. He looked at me. I was shaking in spasms like I did the year before while giving birth.

"Why are you shaking?"

"I'm cold, so cold."

It was the truth, I was so very cold. It must have been the right answer because he gave me his jacket to cover myself. I started babbling, "I respect you so much for overcoming your military troubles and being so strong." I had been a chatterbox at two and it had earned me kudos with the adults in my life. Would it work again?

"Will you see me again, give me your phone number," he said. "You're a nice girl."

"Yes, of course, thank you, thank you so much." I was surprised I could speak. I learned then, that fear has a smell and a taste; like a rotting corpse.

I gave him a fake phone number and even tried to act "normal".

Just then, Linda and her date came back from their "walk", her clothes in disarray. She was chatty and giggly as usual, so my silence didn't arouse suspicion. I even tried to contribute, "Tjadar was good tonight, wasn't he?" Linda gave them the directions to my neighborhood in Brooklyn.

When we arrived a few blocks from my apartment building I spoke, "We're home you can let us out, thanks."

Linda opened her mouth to protest, I gave her a look that stopped her mid sentence. "Happy birthday," Carlos called out as we exited the car.

I shouted "run" and took off my heels like hookers do when the police come and ran for my life. When we entered the lobby of my apartment building, I started punching Linda with both fists and kicked her to the ground.

"You caused this, I said over and over. He hurt me and you caused this."

I didn't know the word "rape", but my anger was huge as I pummeled her. I soon fell to the ground weak and defeated. As was common in New York, some people looked out of their peep holes and proceeded to mind their own business. We entered my apartment and Linda screamed when I took off my tight vest.

"You're bleeding all over," she sobbed.

Had I been knifed? My body had numerous horizontal cuts. The back of my neck had the deepest one, and I remembered the knife pressed against it throughout the attack. The knife was the elephant in the car and I knew if I mentioned it I would die. I just know that. What I'll never know is if he intended to cut me or it happened while he was bouncing on me holding the knife. I entered a steaming tub of water and cried with pain as the wounds sprang to life. The cut on the back of my neck continued to bleed, but after the bath Linda put pressure on it and it stopped. We put iodine on all the cuts and Linda put me to bed with my pajamas and my daughter's teddy bear. Her "I'm sorry, I'm sorry" put me to sleep like a mantra.

I never once thought of going to the police. I couldn't tell this story to anyone. How stupid of me to let this happen. I was always told I made bad decisions and would suffer the consequences, so the attack seemed almost justified. I had been taught to avoid the police or make my mother upset. No man would want me again. I was unclean and my whole existence depended on disproving I was not hideous like my mother constantly hammered into my brain. It was my entire fault because I was so very stupid! I didn't fight him off or scream so the sex must have been consensual. Wasn't it?

I rationalized to make my guilt bearable. In the back of my mind I knew some other unlucky woman would be next. But I had learned at an early age to forget bad things.

In fact, I put the whole experience out of my mind for years. I went to therapy for panic attacks and didn't mention the assault to any therapist. It was only when the attacks got so bad that I was passing out in the middle of streets and became known to the Emergency Medical Technicians (EMT's) by first name that I tried to confront my past. I had never forgotten that night, but thought it was better not to remember. I chose to remember any good that happened in my life after that night, not realizing until much later, that night would come back to poison any good and leave me in a state of endless fear. I never thought that by not confronting anything or anyone, my secret would seethe into the bowels of my soul, arising to attack me again and again.

Many psychologists later, I was almost convinced I was not dirty or evil. The professionals told me I was strong enough at nineteen to save my life; and to understand that night was a perfect storm of Linda's frugality, my conflict avoidant personality and a chance collision with a psychopath.

But, by then, I felt unworthy to have been spared. In insightful moments I realized I had used my intuition to survive evil in a killing mood, and lived because I thought "Cogito ergo sum" (I am thinking therefore I still exist). I had sensed that if I treated a barbarian like a king he might keep me alive. Since it worked that night, I would repeat this behavior in all my future relationships. Many times, I think of another ending, I'm dead and lying in some brush near the car and Linda returns and asks for me. "She ran away when I tried to kiss her," he lies. Maybe Linda would be killed next if she asked too many questions. More likely, she in her evil innocence is driven home to wait for the friend that never returns.

I almost wish I could blame the panic attacks and agoraphobia that plagued my life on the obscenity of that night, but the truth is much darker and started long before that small death.

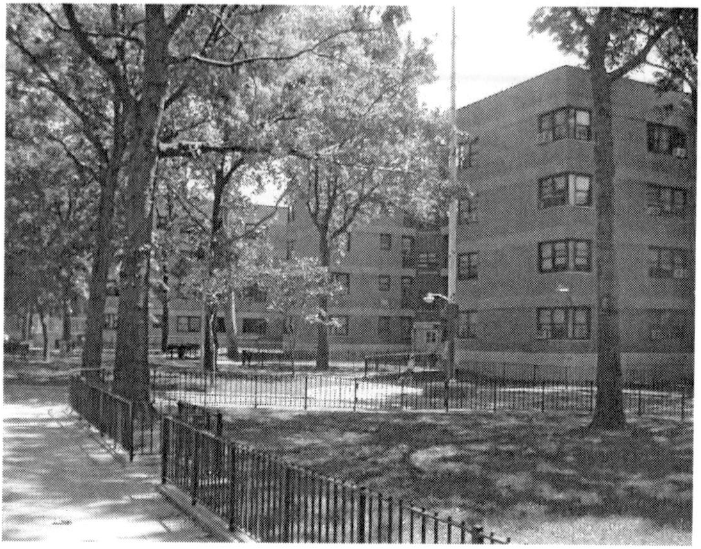

CHAPTER 2

Williamsburg; not Virginia

On June 24, 2003, The Williamsburg Houses was designated a New York City Landmark, comparable to the Chrysler Building and Grand Central Station. I moved there in 1954 at the age of four and even then, I knew it was special. The circular room lay out from the kitchen around to the living room separated by foyers fascinated me as much as the country-like setting.

The first day we moved in I said, “So many doors,” and wandered around in a daze opening and closing them.

“There are twenty doors mommy,” I said as she smiled her rare smile that brought me joy because I'd caused it. I played train in the long foyer near the front door when my mother cleaned the kitchen floor. Lining the chairs back to back, I was both the conductor and the passenger acting out the variety of characters who inhabited my project world.

What I learned later, was the project's overseer was Richard H. Shreve, an architect who worked on the Empire State Building. The head designer, William Lescaze was a Swiss born designer obsessed with the European Modernist style and was determined to bring it to the United States. This style, later called Art Deco was first introduced at the Paris Exhibition of 1925.

Elegantly modern, it reminded me of the Fred Astaire movies I would add to my obsessions in my twenties. Four acres of tan brick four story buildings decorated with blue panels and doorways covered with aluminum marquees became the most progressive and biggest housing project in Brooklyn; advanced and different from the large red brick housing projects set back from patches of skimpy lawn that represented the time.

The time was 1938, and twelve slum blocks depicted in the book, "A Tree Grows in Brooklyn" would be raised. The people living in the cold railroad flats, a series of rooms connected to each other in a line similar to a railway car would now have hot water, steam heat, free electricity and safety.

But back then in 1939, in the architectural journal "Pencil Points," author and architect Talbot F Hamlin said of the Williamsburg Houses,

"It offers more of the amenities of good housing that many Park Avenue apartments lack, in air, in light, in green and growing in humanity and decency."

In 1950, my parents lived on the Jewish South Side of Williamsburg. My grandfather Samuel Chalfin had secured an apartment for my mother in an all Jewish building through his contacts at the local Synagogue. My mother then unofficially changed my father's Puerto Rican name from Carmelo to Carl, and his blue eyes and white skin allowed him to come and go without much religious tension. She asked him not to speak in public because he had an accent similar to Ricky in "I love Lucy." But I'm sure my father's thunderous voice let all the tenants know they had an imposter in their midst. They should have been more afraid of my mother. True to form, she was the last tenant to leave the tenement at 306 Rodney Street. She said living in an empty tenement with mice hiding in her shoe, and the city threatening her with at least jail, only made her more stubborn to stay. Yet all alone in the deserted tenement with powerful men on a mission to build the Brooklyn Queens Expressway was no job for a woman in those days, even my mother. One day they brought in a cop on the beat who stood in the corner with a night stick, while the other men persuaded her to give into the inevitable and leave. As a consolation prize, she was promised a prime four room apartment in the projects;

the Williamsburg Houses, the third and the most expensive project ever made in New York.

Lescaze had tilted the buildings fifteen degrees from the street grid to catch the sun and breezes, creating cross ventilation and when we opened all the doors, it proved an allay to the muggy New York summers. When we looked out the windows we were surrounded by nature complete with trees, squirrels and birds. At 5p.m., the birds would start singing, "What is that noise mommy?" I asked.

"The birds are going to sleep," she said. The birds went to sleep almost as early as I did. I watched Lassie at 7p.m. and after that it was off to bed. Mommy would pat my back until I fell asleep in her bed. I fortunately wasn't privy to the demons that kept her up all night but I was curious about the tell tale signs of her binging left on the thick grey windowsills.

"Who left the crackers, shells, and fruit pits there?" I asked.

"The birds," she answered and I believed her. I slept in her bed until I was eight. She wasn't overly affectionate but showed me more attention than anything, except her books and crackers.

I see myself jumping up and down on our bed. On the bounce up I see white flakes falling from the sky and I ask, "What is that mommy, are there diamonds in the sky?"

My mother mumbles, "Snow." She is sitting by the window plucking her eyebrows in front of the magnifying mirror set up on the windowsill. "Be quiet, I have to put on my face."

"Mommy, you already have a face," I reply, and that remark elicits a half smile as it did when I asked her why she had feathers under her arms. I love Mommy and Mommy loves me. I'm sure. She later told me when I was a baby, she called the doctor because I never cried.

The doctor climbed five flights of stairs before saying, "There's nothing wrong with your baby, she's just happy."

She didn't believe him because happiness wasn't in her vocabulary so she kept looking for something wrong until she found it. But that would be later. Then, I was her wunderkind, her change of life baby. She loved me and she was my world, bigger than life, mesmerizing, and only frightening to other people.

We had a ritual before going to bed. I would lie down next to her and she would gently pat my back until I fell asleep. I was safe next to Mommy. I was a sound sleeper and never awoke until morning. I adored her and my obedience pleased her. Her huge presence kept me safe.

I didn't know we were poor or that my father was disgusted with my mother for leaving her job when she gave birth to me and left her five dollars on the kitchen table for everything except the rent. He was punishing her for not giving him money to open up a restaurant. She punished him by managing to live on the five dollars. Mommy was a true depression era child and had saved five thousand dollars working for the city as a typist and wasn't about to reward my father for his philandering. I was unaware of this drama and only knew I lived in a leafy oasis in the middle of a city. The project was a world in itself with alleys and hideaways that became my playground.

If there were chinks in the amour, I only sensed a few discord notes, like when mommy followed me around outside with a glass jar full of milk. The other kids called me a baby and laughed at my short dresses and chubby thighs but I didn't understand meanness then.

Somehow, I did know it was wrong to pick up the green peppers on the ground of the Italian fruit stand on Grand Street, but mommy said, "the peppers on the ground are free and left there for kids to pick up, if you don't you'll waste them."

I obeyed, but the start of the panic I would carry around like a heavy suitcase for the rest of my life started then, trying to hide my crime from the stern Italian owner. I was too smart to believe I wasn't a thief, but not smart enough to know if I was caught I might be hauled off to jail. Anyway she said she really needed those peppers to make our dinner palatable and my mission was to keep mommy happy. I would hold my breath while I crawled on the floor not looking above until I held the dreaded pepper in my hand and gave it to mommy.

I also knew my legs hurt when we walked five miles to the matzoth factory to get all the broken matzos we could carry for a few cents. I never complained and always smiled what mommy called "the smiling face" and talked to everyone we met. Mommy taught me to recite poetry at two and read by three. I think she was proud of me then. Sometimes, I asked for a toy I saw on TV, but, she just laughed until I did. Later, I begged for cutouts when I learned about the stories you could tell with paper dolls, and she said ok, because they were cheap. My cousin Cindy had the prize Lennon Sisters cutout book, and when I slept over, I pressured her to play. I loved Kathy, the plainest of the sisters and dressed her in the best dress I could wrangle away from Cindy whose favorite sister was Janet, the youngest. The best part was making up stories to go with each dress change. I felt like I was floating in a glorious fantasy world when we did that. I wanted to be there forever. I was always pressuring Cindy to play when I slept over, and I convinced her most of the time, but she wasn't as infatuated with cutouts as I was.

Sometimes a neighbor, surprised I didn't have a real doll brought me one and my world soared as I played with an almost living breathing toy. I didn't understand why mommy always looked sour about it.

One day, I innocently told my mother's friend, "My mommy says you're crazy" and as my mother feebly denied it, the lady sadly said, "I know." Afterwards when mommy got angry, I didn't understand what I had done wrong and to her credit she accepted that children always tell the truth.

I recited "The night before Christmas" at three to all of mommy's friends and Mrs. Berkowitz; a huge woman who smelled like old clothes and urine, gave me apples. I just smiled and put them in my pocket. I never told her I choked on apples if mommy didn't peel them first. I gagged when mommy told me to just chew them harder.

All the project ladies thought I was an angel because I truly was interested in listening and talking to them. This trait would later prove both a gift and a curse.

Big Minnie and little Minnie, my mother's friends fed me matzoth Brei (Jewish French toast) because I didn't run around or yell like other kids. Yetta, who was also crazy according to mommy, had once owned a candy store, and made real chocolate malteds in a stainless steel blender. I remember her taking out the piece of malt from its hiding place and saying to me, "This is what makes it malted milk." I loved them all. I missed them when they all moved to Long Island when the local synagogue went broke. I thought we would move too, but my mother was unmovable in every way, declaring the projects were our forever home.
"Make the best of it," she said.

She then cautiously made friends with the remaining Italian and Black families. Miss Willie Mae was an always laughing three hundred pound single mother of five children who lived on the first floor of our building. Debra, the only girl of five boys was my classmate and friend. One day, while my mother was enjoying her favorite Southern dishes, fried chicken and collard greens in their kitchen, there was an unknown drama to her in the living room. Debra's brothers were curious what naked white asses looked and felt like, so Tommy Taylor told me to take my clothes off and we all marched in a line, while they touched my butt to all our delights. The pleasure ended with one shrill scream when my mother came in to check on me. She stopped all such fun games thereafter, to my disappointment. We never again went to Miss Willie Mae's house but I learned that being in the limelight with boys touching me was pleasurable.

When mommy was in a good mood, or to cajole me to eat, she would play my favorite game "pretend." I was in love with my favorite TV show character, "Brave Eagle." Mommy would be the handsome Indian and I would be Morning Star, his best friend Smokey's daughter.

"How are you today, Morning Star?" she would say.

"Oh dear Brave Eagle, I'm fantastic today," I giggled, batting my eyelashes because at that moment mommy really was Brave Eagle and I was an Indian Princess and that felt so very good. Life with mommy in the projects was wonderful until it wasn't. And it was all because of my father's closet, or was it?

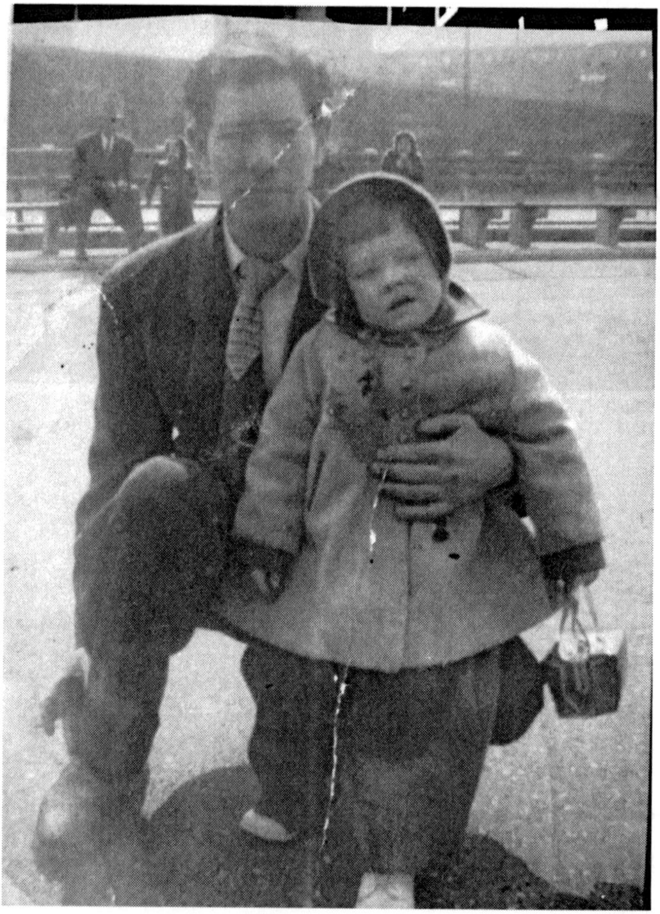

CHAPTER 3

A BOX FALLS ON MY HEAD

My mother had agoraphobia before the disorder was officially recognized. She always became "sick" before any important family gathering. This meant I went to my cousin's big fat Jewish wedding, engagement party, and even the World's Fair in 1963 with my mostly absentee father. Despite my father's frantic juggling of his women, jobs and partying, if my mother really impressed upon him that he should take her place, he was more than ready for a celebration. I would be his date tonight and my face was hot with excitement as I dressed for the evening.

This time it was my Cousin Louise's engagement party. Daddy was as out of place as a pork pie at a Bar Mitzvah. No one understood his thick Spanish accent or attempted to engage him in conversation but he still danced with as many women who couldn't resist his Latin persuasion. He also enjoyed the open bar more than he should have. When it was time to leave he was weaving toward the car, which of course wouldn't start. After a few tries, he turned to me and slurred, "Marilyn you start it." He gave me the keys and I nervously turned the ignition. It started! We both were amazed and his praise filled the empty parts of me at his first real acknowledgement of my presence.

At the 1963 New York's World's Fair my mother again pleaded illness, so my father escorted me. He never complained as we stood in lines for hours to see exhibits and rides he couldn't care less about. He let me go through the "Parker Pen Pavilion" three times to secure the names of pen pals from Denmark, Spain, and Japan. I was in heaven at the process of actually being given a friend who supposedly was hand picked for me.

Going out with my father was a high point of my childhood. I was afraid of most things; the dark, heights, witches, and getting lost. When my father made an appearance in my life, life was good, fun and exciting. I didn't know then about his secret life and I believed his story that he was caring for his mother when he was away. He loved women and lived to charm them out of their drawers.

What he failed to do was protect me. When he witnessed my mother yelling or hitting me, he feebly said, "Leave her alone already."

"Shut up Cahl," she would yell back her usual impeccable diction reverting back to the disappearing New York "R's."

If he was home during her violent onslaughts he would tell me privately. "Try to get along with your mother, don't make her mad." This was impossible and he knew that and should have done something, anything.

The first time he let me down big time was when my mother had her major "nervous breakdown" when I was eight. Her mother Lena had died and she couldn't cope with her grief.

He couldn't resist the thousand dollars my mother put in his pocket to hire a nanny for me, and instead took me to my grandmother's house where no English was spoken. He had his double life to attend to. He did buy himself a shiny new Buick. I call this period, "My father gets a new car and I get screwed."

His most unusual betrayal was an evening I was bored and snooped in his closet, which was in my room, and a box of pornography fell on my head. I was nine and the box was huge. After putting an ice cube on the bump, I opened the box and my heart started pounding. I couldn't stop staring at the images that I didn't understand but somehow knew would be important in my life. When he wasn't around which was most of the time, I escaped to my room as quickly as I could and versed myself on all things sexual. I thought of boys constantly and wanted to practice my new found lessons.

My father visited us on Monday through Wednesday, his long time mistress getting the other half of the week, the good half. My sister Carol calls it "alternate side of the street parking." His excuses for his constant absence, which my mother accepted but was too smart to believe, involved his two sons from his long common law marriage in Puerto Rico. I loved Nestor and Angie, my half brothers, and I fantasized I gave up my father so they could have a better life. But I found out later he was as absent a father to them as he was to me. The only good thing he did for them was taking them away from their alcoholic mother and giving them a ticket to New York. He later sent for my grandmother in Puerto Rico to care for them as my mother would have none of that.

One night she used the "N" word and said,"They're too dark to pass." That was the only time he pushed her against the wall.

My father was not crazy. I say this emphatically, because some people thought him odd to say the least. His life revolved around fun, sex and woman and how he could enjoy all three while being married. I am the only legitimate child of seven children and only because my mother mentally ran circles around him. She got pregnant with me and told him on Monday she wanted to get married but no matter what she would have the baby.

He called on Thursday and said, "You win." She married him but she didn't win.

Daddy had a phone in the closet. He slept in our huge living room and the phone would ring while we watched "The Twilight Zone." He would giggle and put his finger to his lips and enter the closet speaking Spanish that could be heard all over the house. He stayed in that closet for hours flirting and cajoling his many lady callers with his charm. Maybe that's when I learned a locked closet could be a refuge. My mother stayed in her room with her books and television blaring seemingly oblivious to my father's shenanigans. According to him they hadn't slept together or had sex since the first year of their marriage.

But one day, while he was telling this story to his friends, my mother opened her locked door and shouted "liar" and closed it again.

Saying my father's voice was unusually loud would not give his voice it's booming due. If he was hyper happy or hyper angry which were his only two emotions, I put cotton in my ears to lower the volume. I still can't stand loud noise unless I cause it.

One day when he was cooking, he mistakenly reached for the bleach instead of the oil.

When he realized his mistake, the whole building was notified "Ay Dios Mio!" he wailed, hitting his chest and crying. A normal person would have reacted, expecting death or at least pestilence but my mother never flinched or looked up from her book. She knew him well because a few minutes later he was singing his favorite song, in his pleasant singing voice, "My heart cries for you."

When he was home, he slept with a pillow he called his girlfriend, tucked under him and made me laugh. He towel dried my long blonde hair and with my head between his strong legs, I felt safe and loved if only for that moment. We even sometimes played a game which I made up, where we would pick a letter and write all the first names we could think of with the letter. He always won. I was surprised but proud until I found a book in his infamous closet that had every name in the world. Maybe he thought up that game, I knew then how a snake charmer feels when bitten. Yet, when I combed his hair and he purred like a contented kitten I felt needed. My mother never mentioned his indiscretions. Her method of punishment would be to pick at him until he exploded with anger. She hated his happiness more than his cheating.

Then with a small smile she would say, "Close the door Marilyn." I would later determine this was their sex life.

When I was a teenager, on Mondays through Wednesdays, he would put on Salsa, Pachanga and Merengue music and entertain my friends. If I was lucky, he would hold me in his elegant embrace in a slow bolero dance. I was just close enough to inhale his aroma of cologne and cigar and I knew then why he succeeded in the love department.

His favorite program was Benny Hill, a British comedian who acted naughty and crude with women but his real TV obsession was "The Iris Chacon show." Iris Chacon was a Puerto Rican woman as beautiful as the many Miss Universes' that Puerto Rico has contributed, with one big difference. She had an ass as big as her skimpy outfits were small and danced it off to the delight of my father and a continent of drooling Latin men. Thanks to her, I never found my own large behind to be a detriment; until it was pointed out to me by non-Latinos.

And then there was the Christmas day when daddy appeared like a drunken Santa Claus with a load of presents and a tree; which my mother had warned him not to do. We were Jewish she said.

But that day he defied her and said, "The kid deserves Christmas."

He was gone in a flash before she could say anything. I still remember the presents, a Spanish Flamenco doll, and "Ten games in one," which included checkers, chess and Parcheesi. The best prize of all was a real bunny in a carriage. I dressed the bunny and kissed him all night. He had literally pulled a rabbit out of a hat. My father was magic. However the magic included making the bunny disappear with him by morning.

One day he appeared with a puppy I promptly named Floppy for his long ears and forlorn expression. My mother was not pleased but she saw an opportunity to force me to eat huge amounts of food or, "Daddy would take Floppy away." One night while I was in front of what seemed like a thousand potatoes, my mother announced I wasn't eating fast enough and she made my father pick up Floppy and fake take him out to the incinerator, where we burned garbage.

I said, "No, no," and somehow ate all the potatoes and daddy brought him back.

I threw up that night and my mother made my father really take Floppy away. I cried so hard when daddy picked up Floppy, but, for once out of character, I became angry or brave and grabbed one end of Floppy from my father and we started pulling him in opposite directions. We had what could be called "a Puerto Rican standoff" for a few moments but when I heard Floppy cry out, I let go and collapsed on the floor in despair. Daddy had a sad look in his eyes but he couldn't bend to the power that was my mother. I would look for the love that I had with Floppy in that one week my whole life with men who couldn't come close to that dog's affection. I also learned my father was too busy to care about me; he had his own double life to attend to.

The most impressive lesson I learned was that to be accepted by my father or any boys, I would have to be pretty and learn all the secrets in those books and photos.

If I didn't, I would suffer the same fate as my mother and be left alone. In time this would evolve in an obsession with sex and end with boxes that would comfort and house me in my dark hours in closets.

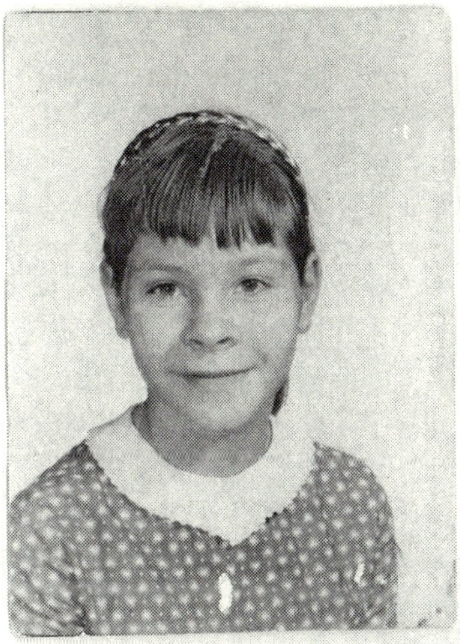

CHAPTER 4

A WAY WITH WORDS

When I was nine, my mother won a contest in the "New York Daily News" putting me down.

"Messy Marilyn Makes Messes, Making Mother Mad." I was young but felt a strange new emotion- pride for her and shame for me mixed up in a big stew of shit.

My mother was prolific in her insults, sarcastic, smart and scary. When she was manic, the words of darkness were screamed in my ear and branded in my soul.

Slop job! Pimple face, bastard, cock eyed, (referring to my lazy left eye) or her favorite "Spotted terrier." To give her credit, she never said the word fuck. But my life was fucked up by words. She was crazy. Not in the funny eccentric mild way of taking to her bed, though she did that too, but in the street lingo of "cuckoo". My father said she had been in every mental ward of every hospital in New York City. I always knew where to find her when I was old enough to enter the scary locked wards. She was the one with the book, always. She was brilliant, a singer, a voracious reader, and she loved me to pieces. I almost fell to pieces. I was her life, however her life was hell.

There were other words as well, words that have stayed with me even though she's now gone. "Cleanliness is next to godliness," she chanted as she burned my face with boiling water twice a day. She had the best intentions. She, along with others, believed dirt caused pimples. When I winced as the boiling water hit my face, she yelled "Ungrateful bastard" both our faces beet red.

Every month we trekked to Manhattan to the "New York University of Skin and Cancer." I loved that place. It smelled rich, from the shiny polished reception area where my mother paid twenty five dollars-CASH, to the empty private waiting rooms where magazines with homes so large, I lived in them in my mind, lie on art deco tables. I belonged there, but my mother clearly didn't and this was proved beyond a doubt one sunny appointment morning.

The doctor, my mother and I were in the room, the final room akin to an audience with the pope. He looked at my eager face and kindly said. "So, how have you been this month?" When I opened my mouth to speak, my mother started a long spiel about her hard work in keeping my face clear.

He looked at her dead in the eye and said, "Madam, I was talking to your daughter." I was so shocked that someone so important thought I was someone worth listening to and more amazed that he silenced my mother; I could only mumble a few words with my head half down, before my mother interjected, but he continued looking at me. Was he sorry for me, did he care? It didn't matter. I was a person to him.

I was always given the same remedy for the cystic acne that plagued me since I was eight years old. Tetracycline antibiotics, Fostex soap and a chalky makeup, we called "stuff." It made me look like a ghost, and smelled and looked ghastly but I always obeyed when she screamed. "Put your stuff on," after she boiled my face. I couldn't swallow the pills due to my throat closing, but mommy had an ingenious plan to deliver this medicine - baby food. She opened the capsules and the disguised round rainbows were blended into applesauce. If I hesitated one moment, because the concoction was bitter, she would yell, "Ungrateful bastard, I'm trying to make you look like a human being," not having clear skin and scars ruined my life. She called the taunting "constructive criticism." Both of my parents had acne and scars, but the genetics of this condition were not known yet, she knew somehow she was guilty about this and other secrets she kept and it made her hate both of us for my condition. Mom hand fed me until I was twelve. I couldn't get away from the two food items, I still can't forget, a baby cereal called "Pablum" and a soft boiled egg.

According to Wikipedia, Pablum is a processed cereal for infants marketed by the "Mead Johnson Company" in 1931. It is also used metaphorically especially in literary criticism to refer to something bland and unappetizing. I was forced to eat Pablum cereal and the almost raw egg until I was twelve. Mommy told me I threw up the first five years of my life. I only remember walking up the elevator train steps one by one it seemed toward a skewed heaven. At the top, overcome with vertigo my stomach would release its contents.

I still have a hard time holding utensils without dropping them. Doctors have told me it is a combination of delayed motor skills and anxiety. I am notorious for falling down in every city or town I've ever been in. My sister Carol calls me "a disaster waiting to happen."

I made a board of psychiatrists utter a collective gasp by telling them I was hand fed by my mother until puberty. When the door closed after me, the chatter I heard in the room made me feel like a fool for revealing my shameful secrets. I never doubted ma loved me. I doubted I was worth loving.

I was her change of life baby and she would do right by me, if it killed both of us which it almost did. One of her psychiatrists in her last years told me it took a special combination of art and intellect to insult people like my mother did. I made a promise that day to stay stupid.

"How can you be so vulgar and shameful to wear a uniform with a spot on it? She had scolded a nurse during the last days of life.

"We made up," she said later, but knowing how she could inspire hatred. I actually thought her sudden death had been advanced by her "way with words".

There were other words that were even more damaging to my tenuous self-esteem.

"You're too ugly for anyone to want to ever marry you," her face twisted with hate as she ran after me to pinch my arms until they were bruised or pull my long hair until it came out in clumps in her hands.

Someone will marry me I'll show you, I thought and even surprised myself when I wore an engagement ring at sixteen. The down side was that my apprentice with the master taught me to accept abuse and unpredictable people. Evil senses weakness and I was easy prey.

Eventually, I stayed in my room as much as possible and found out I was relatively safe there. I realized my room was a place where words couldn't hurt me.

When I turned fourteen and rebelled, she used her nails to scratch me as she challenged my self-esteem with words that hurt worse than the sticks and stones she said wouldn't break my bones. I was the human that had come out of her and she wanted me to be what I couldn't be; perfect. She wasted a lot of money and time trying to find the miracle elixir to clear my acne which was just as incurable as the mental illness she tried to hide. I heard the words "shock treatments" and "loony bin" whispered around me, hoping I wouldn't catch her "sickness."

I found out later there's a worse scarring that no amount of crushed pills can remedy. It's the scarring of the soul and I knew I had to leave her presence as soon as I had the chance. Call it the words of my being, my higher power, an inner child that wouldn't be destroyed by words.

CHAPTER 5

THOMPSON

I always knew I would run away from home but in 1955, my passport was my library card and my destination was the "Devoe Street Library" in Brooklyn. How I loved that place. First of all, it was quiet. You had to be quiet. What a concept! Since my house was bedlam; literally, I thought it was astonishing that there were people who were silent on purpose. The red brick building would become my refuge. I loved the librarian with her tight bun and quiet voice. I always made sure I had an important question to ask her when I shyly approached. And what was important, no; vital to my then six-year-old self was fairy tales. Grimm's and Hans Christian Anderson became my escape from a life I somehow knew was not right. I was a child; I didn't understand, poverty, chaos, even abuse in the grown up way. I just knew reading made everything better.

I walked to the library by myself even though it was at least a half mile from my house. What an odd sight I must have made. I have a lazy left eye or as it is medically known now, Strabismus. I wore glasses, had white blonde hair with the uneven bangs cut by my father, and carried my allotted four books piled high near my nose. I was tall for my age, but the books were so heavy that my glasses always slid off my nose. They still do.

When I entered the hall to go up the stairs, the familiar comforting figure of Thompson, the projects Colored porter stood, leaning on his mop, saying hello to someone. I always said, "Hi Thompson," like everyone did.

He always stopped, looked me in the eyes like I was important to him and said, "Hello baby." Often when I arrived home he was sitting with my mother in the kitchen, on his break, his mop against the wall as he bent close to my mother gossiping over coffee. I drank in his kind brown eyes and quiet presence. It was a respite, a soothing compress to my sore head. When Thompson appeared, I knew my mother would be in a good mood. He treated me like I was his daughter, and I wanted to be his daughter.

Thompson was always fixing something and chatting with the housewives. He enjoyed my mothers witty remarks and seemed engrossed in her stories about how this or that neighbor was a tramp and fooling around with someone's husband or how one woman named Mrs. Kaplan was "nuts" and should be avoided. I always knew I was safe if Thompson was there because mommy was happy. I walked into my room with my treasures and entered my fairy tale world. I was Rapunzel and letting down my golden hair to be let out of my tower, or Snow White, but I wasn't alone, I had a sister; Rose Red, who was my confidante, my friend. I hardly noticed when Thompson left the house and my mother started screaming,

"Look at your face; you can cut the grease with a knife."

I knew It was time for the boiling water.

I hardly noticed when the water attacked my face. I didn't resist, not because my hair would be pulled, but I was a princess who was protected from such plebian activities. I had my castle. I had my books, and I had Thompson.

If I were to see him today, I would thank him for being my part time protector, a father figure, and the real king of my imaginary kingdom. Most of all, I would tell that now I now know his name was Mister Thompson and I wish with all my heart, I had been taught that.

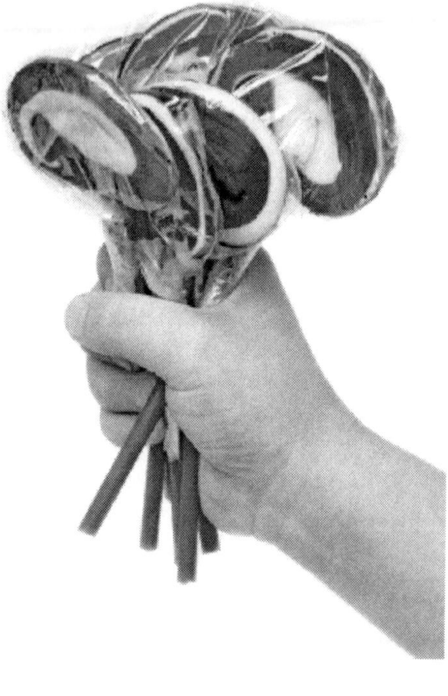

CHAPTER 6

OFFER THEM CANDY

I had a bad habit of marrying anyone who asked me. Of course he had to have a list of qualities which has nothing to do with husband suitability, like speaking two languages, driving a stick shift, and Salsa dancing like a champion. He also had to be won over before he despised me. As you can imagine, this approach has not served me well. I blame this on my kindergarten experience.

I had a crush on Jimmy DeWitt, a tan, dimpled curly haired hunk to be. My rapt attention must have turned him off as much as it did to the many other men who would inhabit, then disappear in my life. He started bullying me and my adoration turned to fear; also familiar in my life. He would then growl and threaten to do me bodily harm. Again, familiar. I was afraid to leave the house to go to school, then work, ok, familiar.

My mom had the answer. She bought a "lollipop bouquet," a treat I was rarely allowed and told me to offer a few pops. The next day, averting my eyes, I held out my prize to Jimmy. He grabbed the whole treasure and smiled, all his dimples working. Hey, I thought, I wanted the cherry one. Although he never gave me trouble the rest of the year, I felt a certain emptiness and depression that would also become a well established part of my future.

Miss Andersen, the kindergarten piano teacher was an ageless, mentally absent woman who shared her job with Miss Lansky, a young blonde cheerleader. I worshipped them. My favorite part of the day was when Mrs. Anderson played the piano and we all took turns trotting in a circle. The girls chose boy partners and even though I was shy I picked Jimmy. When he accepted and held my hand my love of dance and boys began. I never chose Jimmy again after the candy incident, selecting instead a skinny boy who never smiled and cried when his mother left. My least favorite time also evolved during that school year.

Three times a week, the class was assigned instruments and we played to songs like “She’s coming around the mountain” and “I’ve been working on the Railroad.” The excitement started as Mrs. Anderson handed out the drums, horn, and cymbals to the boys. (This was the fifties). The girls were offered the daintier silver accompaniments, like the flute, clarinet, and my dream, the triangle.

The triangle: a dream of brass shiny loveliness had a little implement which made a delightful tinkle when struck. Inevitably, I was given two wooden sticks. They made a hollow noise and brought to my little mind uselessness and unprettyness. I hated those damn sticks. Throughout the year, I waited with anticipatory hope that the triangle or later, any other instrument would come my way. I was always disappointed. The sticks became my enemy. I was given them week after week I wanted to stomp on them or throw them at Michelle, the girl who was offered the triangle week after week. I didn’t eat crayons like Ramona or pee on the floor like Selena. What about me said sticks? Yet, every day I would hope against hope that I would be given something else. It never happened. I was stuck with the sticks.

After music time, I finger-painted with joy, forgetting any frustration. I dipped my fingers in pots of rainbows smearing wiggly lines on rough paper. I always exited the door with a wide smile.

My mother always said the same thing. “Why are you always the only one with a dirty face?”

I looked around and it was true. However, there was one comfort waiting for me at the entrance of the school. I had a classmate named Ernest whose mother was blind. She had a Seeing Eye dog, named Rusty. Our mothers always waited for us at the school's entrance, and though the blind mother rarely spoke, she created a calm demeanor that made an impression on me. No one was allowed to play with the dog when he was working but I always felt happy when I saw him. One day, she spoke to me after my mother's usual comment. Marilyn, why don't you pet Rusty? He knows you already." Her voice had such a gentle tone it made me wish she was my mom and I could be with Rusty forever. I gently stroked his rough skin and he looked up at my dirty face with love in his warm brown eyes. I felt a sense of peace and unconditional love, a first for me, and would thereafter seek that in my life unsuccessfully with false friends and unworthy men.

I gave myself away with that bunch of lollies and was left with an empty wrapper and two worthless wooden sticks. But the most dangerous lesson I learned in kindergarten was allowing people to mistreat me. I don't know why I was never given the triangle, but my childlike trust in people was never completely crushed. If all else failed, I offered them candy.

CHAPTER 7

SHE TAKES THE CAKE

My mother told me I hated cake. I was the only kid at the birthday party who didn't eat the cake. I did eat vanilla ice cream because I was told I liked it. I could only have it in a cup because I was a "slop job" and couldn't handle a Popsicle properly. I was also told I didn't like broccoli because my mother hated it. We had the typical 50's diet with an atypical way of eating. First of all, my father always propelled his food, without asking on to my plate. I thought this was normal until I attempted this with my boyfriend Hiroki in Japan forty years later. He went apoplectic but I blamed it on his explosive anger disorder.

Hiroki's son, who was a restaurant manager in Thailand, said he always knew who the Americans were because they rarely used their knives. A knife in our house was only for cutting huge pieces of rare steak, and forks were used to shovel the food almost whole into your gullet as fast as possible.

The menu for lunch featured bean with bacon soup, a bologna or tuna sandwich and salty corned beef hash. I was told I liked those as well. I think I did. What I know I hated for sure was the soft boiled egg and the baby cereal she hand fed me until I was twelve.

I never ate those two food items again and even saying them makes me nauseous. I became smart about avoiding food when I got older. I was not allowed to hang out with my friends until I choked down three huge plain potatoes without even butter to make them palatable. My friends would come and put said potatoes into their pockets and then into the project incinerator. (The project incinerator, though the opposite of green living, was a most excellent apparatus). You watched the flames and inhaled the smoke as you threw your garbage away and every floor had one. You just had to be careful you were not mugged while outside your steel door with the five locks. I used to get nervous when it was my turn. I started feeling like one of those teenagers in a horror film when they find out a guy in a mask is running after them. Those few inches traveling from the heavy project door, opening the heavy chute and slamming the door against all monsters was tortuous.

But when the potatoes were eaten or thrown away, I was allowed to go to St. Mary's Church Friday night Confraternity dance where all the cute Puerto Rican boys were. I learned how to lie and to save myself from my mother's unusual food requests until I was more bold than clever and got caught. My ponytail was pulled so hard; I had a headache for a week.

My mother's wrath was worse than the imaginary monster at the incinerator when she chased me around and around our circular house. I was faster than her but eventually she caught me. Once while chasing me, she broke one of my grandmother's twin cut glass bowels, she had inherited. Her anger was dissipated a little because she knew I loved those two heirlooms as much as she did.

The bowls and a lavender satin comforter brought me joy and were only put on display during our project inspections.

"Daddy waxed the floor," she would say the day the dreaded, to my mother, inspector came.

My mother was always proud when he said, "Mrs. Mendoza, you are in the top five of our cleanest apartments."

The project inspections stopped around the time the welfare workers started getting mugged on their unhappy job of visiting people who didn't want their life inspected.

"Let's see how much dust is in the corners of his house," Della, the neighbor with six kids said to my mother. My mother told me Della always received warnings on her welfare inspections. Once, they found a man hiding in her closet. I couldn't figure out why a man would do that but I was young then.

Food was the beginning of our battles but for me it became my way of being separated from her craziness. Oh, and there was a LOT of craziness. At dinner, especially when my father was home, Monday through Wednesday, my mother took out her anger at his infidelity by pushing him until his explosive anger disorder erupted. Mmm....Well, we didn't know that term then. She complained about the food he would cook to placate her, and call him names though never referring to the actual events that made her so angry. I would feel a lump in my throat and sometimes could not digest the heavy Puerto Rican food he cooked. I knew I had to eat it and then I would get that nervous feeling that made it hard to swallow as I would plot on how the food would get in the incinerator that night. If I didn't eat every crumb, some kid in Europe I never knew would starve. I began to hate those kids and wished there was a way I could smuggle them the food.

There were televisions blasting in every room and since we didn't have to pay for electric in the projects, the light's glared like an unhappy Christmas. I learned to say I had homework which would allow me to escape to my room as soon as possible.

Sometimes we went out to eat "Chinks," I didn't know this was a racial slur until I got older. I thought it meant Chinese food. My father would make fun of the waiter and ask for "flied lice." That was something I knew was wrong, but to tell him would be asking for it, because my mother laughed at the same tired joke every time. I thought I noticed a flicker in the waiters' eyes when my father insulted him, and briefly as the waiters and my eyes met, we looked at each other with sadness and humanness. There was something there that suggested he spoke better English and had a better education than both of my parents.

I was proved correct when I had a long conversation with him when I was sixteen and able to eat in restaurants alone. He was chemistry major in college and spoke perfect English.

My father had a Spanish accent that was not understandable but he was proud of being a white Puerto Rican which made him special in the Puerto Rican culture then. If he wasn't so white it would not have been possible for my Jewish mother to marry him. Even so, she had been a rebel to marry outside the Jewish faith in 1950.

We ate the same meal every time - tomato egg drop soup, chicken chow mein, and pork fried rice, egg rolls and vanilla ice-cream for desert. My father would order shrimp in his chow mein but my Jewish mother didn't eat seafood though inexplicably, she ate pork. We thought we were really eating Chinese food. Now I think how the restaurant owners were laughing at us and had the last laugh because they probably retired to Boca Raton with the money they made off of the "barbarians" who preferred chop Suey to authentic Cantonese dishes.

Once at the same Chinese restaurant, I said, "mom I tried out for the school play "South Pacific" at school." As the waiter approached us with the plate of fortune cookies, she shouted. "You have a "Chinaman's chance" of being picked with that broken out skin of yours.

We all knew (including the waiter) this was not a good chance. My parents were from two minorities, but tolerance was not part of their vocabulary or backgrounds.

To say, my mother hated the Japanese and the Germans would be an understatement. The Japanese were clever and sneaky: re Pearl Harbor and the only good German was a dead German. I later understood why she harbored such hatred about Germans because we lost our family in the Holocaust. She also feared Black people and said most Polish people were Jew haters. Even though she made friends with people from different backgrounds in the projects, she felt more comfortable with the Jewish people who moved to Long Island in the late sixties. Both my parents made fun of each other's cultures and since I am a product of both of them I never felt accepted in either.

Yet, even as a child, I somehow instinctively knew that people have more similarities than differences. When I was three and saw "The March of the Siamese children" in the movie "The King and I" I felt something so powerful that I started crying and lowered my head to hide my tears from my mother; suspecting even then, that my feelings would not be validated; whatever they were.

This movie started my life long obsession with Asian men as well as a small inner rebellion not to be like my parents. I would show them the error of their ways by living my life in a way that was as different from theirs as possible. This proved undoable.

Still, my interest in writing to pen pals impressed my mother enough to read the letters from my pen pal Hiroko Oda a girl from Sapporo Japan. She agreed the girl was kind and maybe she had been too hasty at condemning the whole Japanese race. But In the end her history and upbringing were too strong for her to tolerate my multicultural lifestyle.

I was bowed but not broken and my fear didn't prevent me from making my own decisions; good and bad, she continued to battle me on many fronts. My dieting was "feast or famine."

Since eating in our family was either a battle or an orgy, when I became semi free at sixteen, I developed a love hate relationship with food that lasted for many years. I developed obsessions with different foods and began binging to comfort my fears and anxiety. I was either binging or dieting both done with a ferociousness that scared me. My housecleaning was "lousy cleaning" and she laughed when she saw me reading a book on housecleaning.

"Marilyn is reading a book called 'How to clean house while lying in bed, '" she joked to whoever was present. But since schoolwork was my only chore despite my father's protest that reading was worthless, and my mother had better teach me how to wash and iron like all good Puerto Rican girls; I couldn't win. I was worthless and she wasn't joking. I vowed that when I had children I would never call them names or force them to eat and when they would go to parties, I would let them eat cake.

CHAPTER 8

BLINDED BY THE LIGHT

Prospect Park is a bucolic slice of paradise in Brooklyn New York. It was an escape from the unrestrained bedlam of summers in the projects. In May, when the lilacs were in bloom we also went to the Brooklyn Botanical Gardens. My mother never got tired of the lavender blossoms.

One day when I was seven, Prospect Park became hell for me. I only remember fragments of that day; my mother, her sister Sylvia, and I strolling through the park while my mother cried and cried. My aunt was trying to console her while I bit my lips, so frightened and confused at what was happening.
Now I know the facts of that day. My grandmother, Lena Deborah Chalfin Jaffe had died. Lena my gram, with her soft brown eyes and deep love for me was my mother's rock. She spoke only Yiddish.
"Shana Madala (Pretty girl) she would always say to me. We visited her everyday. I still remember the cups and saucers she had carried in her bag from Russia in the cupboard on South 8th street in Williamsburg. In her last days she suffered a stroke, and my aunt Ethel, who was "slow", would push her around in a chair.

It is the Jewish custom not to talk to children about death, so I only felt my mother's grief that day as a sadness that would stay with me forever. I didn't understand the reason for the darkness, but the anguish; powerlessness and helplessness were very real. I wanted my mother to stop crying that Sunday in the park but she continued at home when my father come home and that's when my so called "normal" life as I had known it went plum loco.

I was taken away from my home a few days later. I was told my mother had a nervous breakdown. That's what they called it then. She was my world. Where would I go? I found out later she had given my father a thousand dollars to find a nanny for me and let me stay home near my school. But a thousand dollars in that time was a fortune and I was sacrificed for a snazzy blue Dodge, and the new girlfriend that came with it.

I was dumped on my other grandma, the Puerto Rican one who also spoke no English and my two half brothers who did. My grandmother, Dona Julia adored me but we also lived with my evil cousin Aurea. She was around twelve, did most of the housework and in her spare time tortured me. I was pinched black and blue, behind my Dona Julia's back. She stuck her tongue out at me and cursed me in Spanish. I think they were curses because although I spoke no Spanish due to my mother's edict, Aurea's face would twist with such hatred I could barely look at her. I offered to help with the dishes, but my grandma told her I was special because I was blonde and blue eyed just like my daddy. My grandma, was "tregena", very tanned, and adored my dad whom I resemble. You can see where this is going.

Aurea got her revenge. Her job was to pick me up after school at 3 p.m. She never came on time. She came later and later and I would tremble when the school bell rang its final death toll. One night I was there until the stars came out and I remember staring at the moon, a small figure near big bridge thinking, "This is the night I will not be picked up." Real fear started that day. I was seven and lost.

I learned the Spanish word for sick the next day, "enferma" and used it as often as I could get away with. I really was sick. I would wake up having to face the ordeal of not knowing if Aurea would pick me up or not. I begged my grandmother to let me stay home and she gave in most of the time because I probably looked as sick as I felt. I later found out Aurea told my grandmother she had taken me to parties, and out for ice cream and that was why we were so late for dinner. I didn't ask my brothers for help because I was too scared, I was afraid they might not like me anymore and I really needed them to like me.

My grandmother was very religious. She was a Pentecostal, which to me meant loud and late. I was this sheltered Jewish girl, who went to bed at 7:30 after Lassie and now midnights found me in the midst of a crazy party. There were tambourines and singing and stout women falling in the aisles and wailing for Jesus. The real "fun" started when they began talking in tongues. I hid my head and imagined I was in my castle but the nightmares and sleepy mornings found me trying to finagle my way out of going to school.

During this time, my father never visited me. I waited and waited to tell him about Aurea, but he was too busy with shiny cars and sex to care about his abandoned daughter. To him I was being taken care of by his mother so what was the problem?

To get some relief from my stress, I acted in front of the dark television, on the rare days I was alone. I had a friend I made up. His name was Mark and he protected me from any problems. He liked me and I became Melanie, my first alter ego, and I poured out my heart, not about the reality of my situation, but how we were in a beautiful castle where silence was valued and where he protected me from ogres and monsters. I would change my voice while playing his part. I felt he was real and almost saw him in the blackness of that dusty television.

My two half brothers were Angel and Jose Nestor. Angel was quite the opposite of his name, and many a night he was chased around the house by my grandmother wielding a broom and screaming at him. Nestor was the golden boy, my father's favorite child. He was friendly and called me "baby." I worshipped him and wouldn't want him to not smile at me or teach me the few words of Spanish that kept me home, so I kept silent about my suffering. They were teenagers and in their own world anyway.

My father didn't come to see me for two months. When he finally arrived to bring me to the hospital to visit my mother, he was dressed in new duds and shined with pride when he introduced me to his "friend" Prima. He joked she was our cousin because prima means cousin in Spanish. I didn't waste time telling him about Aurea, I was no dummy. The mood turned dark for a moment as he translated the news to my grandmother. I can't say I felt sorry when the yelling started and Aurea got a beating.

Then off we went to the hospital. I was not allowed to go up nor were my brothers. So we stood outside a tall building. They were not in the best of moods. What teenagers want to go to hospital on a weekend? I remember standing and being told we were to wait for a signal from my father. My mother was to make an appearance at her window and wave to me. I was short but looked up at the window until my neck hurt. I missed my mother and my life so much. They said, "See, she is there waving at you. Can you see?" I couldn't. I was short, and wore glasses for the weak muscle in my left eye.

"Look up;" they shouted at me, "she's waving." I tried so hard to see her but the building was too tall and I was too short and excited. I kept saying, "where, where?"

Finally Nestor said, "You're the one who put her there, why can't you see her?"

I looked up and was enveloped in a blinding white light. I couldn't' see the building. I couldn't see my brother and most of all I couldn't see my mother. I would be blind for two days and no one would notice while I stumbled around the house.

Again they asked, "Can't you see her?"

I said, "Yes, I can see."

She was so beautiful, only sixteen and the most beautiful girl in our family, even on our block. Her name was Miriam. She was my sister. I couldn't name my daughter after her but I used the first letter as is the way in our religion.

The guilt I feel about her death is a wasted emotion, the therapist said, but my guilt is too big.

She begged me to go to the dance for weeks. She was an "A" student, tall, expressive dark eyes, and she didn't have a bad word to say about anyone. Everyone loved her. Not me, I was a trouble maker and always fought with my father.

I slept with my boyfriend. I was forced to have an abortion on my kitchen table even though I wasn't even pregnant. I'm sure of this. My guilt is not about that, only shame and anger, but my guilt is Miriam. I let her come to the dance. She was so popular and happy that night. I was the only one working at a real job. I was a typist for the city. I gave most of my money to my mother. They needed it. It was the depression, but I wanted nice clothes and the silk blouses that made me somewhat happy like the dances. My angelic mother only said "Another bloose"

Why did I take her out that night? She was always begging me to take her. Why that night? She got sick right after that; scarlet fever and she died very soon after. Heart complications they said, but I knew it was my fault. I got down to 89 pounds, food stuck in my throat and I was never the same after that. I hurt my mother. I was always an angry person, but, after Miriam's' blood was on my hands I became dangerous.

Part 2

IF ONE CAN ACTUALLY REVERT TO THE TRUTH, THEN A GREAT DEAL OF ONE'S SUFFERING CAN BE ERASED---BECAUSE A GREAT DEAL OF ONE'S SUFFERING IS BASED ON SHEER LIES

R.D LAING

CHAPTER 9

DOUBLE DUTCH

"Go, go," I am ten years old and a crowd of mostly young men are gathering around the Williamsburg Projects playground and encouraging me to win the Double Dutch competition.

I believe I am the center of attention because I had been taught by the best colored girls on my team. My heart is beating with excitement and pride; my first taste of fame and I crave it. I naively think it's my skills that are attracting so much attention. I keep jumping without making a mistake, not wanting to let my audience down. On the outskirts, I hardly see the older women looking on disapprovingly.

When I came home, my mother was waiting with her "wait until I get you alone look", but I was so proud of my double dutch prowess, I hardly noticed. A neighbor is explaining to her that she needs to buy me a bra. My bouncing breasts have been inflaming the boys to a feverish pitch. I don't quite understand, but when she leaves I hurriedly speak, "Mom I was the best double dutch player and I helped my team win."

She didn't answer at first, just looked at me with contempt, then she shouted, "They were looking at your bust, you moron." I was dumbfounded and shamed. This would be a familiar sensation in my life, having my enthusiastic naivety rained on by different abusers, changing my joy to deep depression.

My mother was very frugal. She had to be. My father left five dollars on the table and only paid the rent. She had to feed us and do everything else with that money. Bras and sanitary pads were luxuries we could not afford. Since I had my first period so young, she had taught me to attach rags with safety pins to my panties when I got my period. The rags were so huge they bunched up like a mountain under my skirt but yet never seemed to fail soiling my panties.

One day, I came home to her boiling the rags. I said in all innocence, "Fe fi foe fum, I smell the blood of an Englishman," a rhyme I had read in a book.

I really always say the wrong thing, because her nails dug into my hand as she yelled, "You're disgusting and it's a pain in the neck to be your mother."

The dentist who suggested I needed braces really got a tongue-lashing.

"She does not, there's nothing wrong with her teeth, you quack."

Today, I have braces at fifty-nine because my crooked teeth kept biting my tongue. But then, I was terrified of dentists and was happy my mother yelled at the dentist. And my mother was often right in her opinions. I am one of the few of my generation with my tonsils and adenoids because my mother told the doctor she didn't believe in operations, and there was no way I was getting mine out. She was proved right.

The next day after the double dutch incident, she reluctantly took me bra shopping. I had been asking her for a bra since I was nine because the girls in my class who had much less than I, were wearing training bras. I was looked at closely by the Orthodox Jewish man at the discount store where my mother shopped and announced I was a 32A. His sharp eyes turned out to be very accurate.

The next time I jumped rope, the crowd began to scatter as my thick cotton pointy bra kept me as still and invisible as I felt. I heard what would be a constant comment most of my life. "Marilyn has a nice shape but..." At home, it was always my flaws that were pointed out to me, but I began to believe, even though I was a "spotted terrier", my acne was not as important in the eyes of men as my long thick blonde hair and shapely figure. Men would overlook acne and crossed eyes if my body was as good as people said it was.

I was considered a freak at camp when I woke up in the middle of the night with blood gushing. I thought I was dying and Abbey, the plump motherly camp counselor told me I was a lady now and got me a sanitary napkin and also taught me how to use it. However, the other campers were not so easily fooled. They knew how unusual it was for an eight year old to have breasts and a period. They all had flat chests and were small. I was as tall as I would ever be, five feet and one half inch. Even before that incident I was unpopular at camp. I had never been taught to feed or wash myself and taking care of me was a new experience. I was unkempt with my hair a "rat's nest" and my face and hands always dirty. I also fell down all the time, and was so shy I was thought at first to be retarded. I also had nice clothes that were hand me downs from her sister who was four years older and had a figure like mine. I was good at acting, but even now I can't eat without dropping utensils and have fallen more times than I can count.

I was never told about sex then, though it was whispered about in school. Janey, a thirteen year old who was pregnant in Junior High said sex was great and like a rocket blasting off in you. I couldn't see that image without feeling fear, but she was happy so I assumed sex was good, whatever it was.

When I came home from camp, my mother just told me to stay away from boys and if they touched me I would become pregnant, which she assured me was a bad thing. This bad advice would precipitate an incident that caused me to have an early traumatic experience. Alfred, the cute boy next door who was a few years older than me and one of the boys at the double dutch competition, had been a friend since my father had dumped me at his house for a week when my mother had her breakdown when I was seven. We would talk to each other and play music out of our bedroom windows so one day when he knocked on my door when my mother was out, I let him in since he told me he got locked out. Then right there in the long hallway, he grabbed me and held me tight and kissed me. I was horrified. I pushed him away and told him to leave.

With my heart beating fast, I said over and over, "Stupid, I am so stupid, I will get pregnant now. I have really messed up again. Why does everything I do turn out wrong?" That would be a familiar question that would haunt me during most of my life. For seven months, I lived in terror and watched my body to show some signs of pregnancy. I had seen Janey's swollen body so I woke up with fear every morning expecting my body to betray me. I had disobeyed my mother and if she knew there would be hell to pay. In the cloakroom at school I avoided being touched by boys when hanging my coat. I basically lived in fear.

One day, I told Avis, a girl in class who was friends with Alfred that he had kissed me. Alfred had become popular and I wasn't so I wanted Avis to be my friend, to think I was worth her friendship. I made her do the "cross your heart and hope to die" vow, that she would never tell anyone this secret. I never told her my fear of being pregnant because in the seven months since that incident in the hallway my stomach was as flat as ever. The bitch squealed to Alfred, and he denied it ever happened.

"I could never kiss such an ugly pimply face girl," he told her. "She's a liar."

And then to convince her, he yelled it in front of me at our hallway in front of many of the boys who had been watching me jump rope. His words burned my ears as I walked up my stairs. I was mortified and this was betrayal on so many levels. People couldn't be trusted, people lied; people were mean. I retreated into my shell, and never told anyone about the episode.

Despite the shame, I also received another subtle message. I could attract boys and maybe someone would marry me and take me away from this hell of a life. Marriage became my goal at ten, and I would prove my mother wrong. Boys would end up "standing in a line" like the Stevie Nicks song I danced to in the 80's, for a chance to be with me. I had power and the power was called sex. Even if I didn't know quite what it was, I just knew I had "it" and it was powerful. I sensed my father had betrayed me for it, like Alfred had, and the boys in the playground knew I possessed it. I would find out how to be good at it and use it to get a husband and be free. I stopped playing Double Dutch that day.

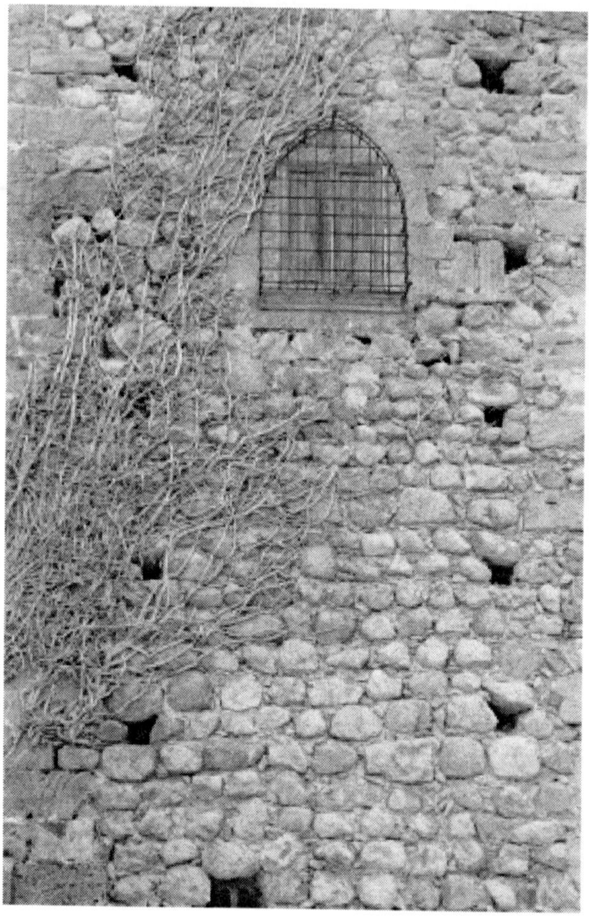

CHAPTER 10

THE PRINCESS AND THE PEA

My first full blown panic attack happened when I was nine at Bear Mountain State Park in upstate New York. I was a day camper with the Williamsburg Community Center located inside my housing project in Brooklyn. After a short tour and lunch, we were given free time to explore the park and told to meet at 4 p.m. I was enjoying the playground with some new playmates when startled; I looked around and could not recognize anyone from my camp. The place seemed distorted and as I looked around, I felt dizzy and my heart pounded so hard I felt it in my head. I started running around trying to find someone. Had they left me like my cousin Aura to fend for myself and find my own way home and where was I anyway? The sense of disorientation made me start running and running. Suddenly Theresa, a girl from our group was in front of me.

"I'm so glad to see you," I said and hugged her. "Did our bus leave?"

"Of course not, she said confidently, I'm still here."

I tried to hug her again but she backed away slightly and smiled. I loved her that moment.

I had other moments of panic before that; small incidents where I would lose my mother in a store or had to climb up high stairs. I was scared of doctors, dentists, and any teachers who were strict. I was especially scared of being called on to be "hall monitor" and my terrified face must have been obvious to the teacher because I never had to do that job the whole year. That didn't stop the panic that welled up in my throat every day she looked around the room to choose someone. I was scared of the dark, monsters, and witches. And most of all, I was scared of Brenda Johnson.

It was the summer of 1959. I had just come back from the camp where I had my first period and thought I was dying. I wasn't allowed to swim in the lake lest I poison the water, so I became the camp outcast. I never learned how to swim and instead of the "sharks" the group where most of the campers graduated to, I would remain a "perch" for the whole four years at Camp Vacamas. I was so afraid of putting my face in that murky lake and drowning. I was also an outcast for being afraid of getting in a rowboat, having a perpetually dirty face and a freak for having breasts and staining my sheets with blood at eight. I came home to a mother who told me not to let a boy touch me or I would get pregnant. This led to another crisis in the future but first I had to deal with Brenda Johnson.

After sleep away camp, my mother sent me to day camp and it was there one day I met my nemesis. Brenda was a colored girl as we said then, and hung out with a group of girls who loved to sing. They entered the camp talent contest, singing "Alley Oop" and though they didn't win, they were so talented and fun, my face held on to my famous smile that always got me in trouble one way or another. I was confronted and surrounded by Brenda and her four friends at the end of the day with the accusation I had laughed at them. I vehemently denied that I had laughed. I said I was smiling because they were so good, and they were the best. I was so sincere; they finally believed me, except Brenda. She sensed that fear in me and that sparked the bully in her. She started threatening me every time she saw me. When I entered the projects I died a thousand deaths before we walked in, so in fear, I refused to look at the benches where the girls hung out.

One summer evening when we were returning from the movie "Some like It Hot," with Marilyn Monroe, Jack Lemmon and Tony Curtis, I momentary forget my tormentor because I was lost in the fantasy of that wonderful movie. She appeared in front of me, like an evil smile in a nightmare. I tried to hide my head into my mother's dress. Ma pushed me off and I hung my head like a camel in the sand, only unlike a camel, I felt deep shame. I should have held my head high in the knowledge no one would harm me in front of my mother but irrational fear held me in its tight grip. During that hot summer, Brenda held the power she had over me like a medal, keeping me plotting not to go out and deal with the bullying.

I was thirteen the first time I ended up in an emergency room. Brenda wasn't the cause; I ended up there because Gerald Washington hated me. He didn't hate me because I was white, he didn't hate me because we had issues. He hated me because I was Chuchie's best friend and they had had a fist fight the week before in front of the whole projects and she had won. He had short and wiry on his side and she had big and burly on hers. He felt he had been humiliated and started picking on someone he could terrorize. That would be me.

We were on the arch, an architecture structure in the projects that was perfect for our teen hangout. There weren't many kids that day because the week before an eight year old girl was raped and thrown off the roof. The roof was also our hangout and like the Drifters song, "Up on the roof," we escaped the summer heat singing and star gazing. But this summer we were forbidden to go out at night and most of the kids were at the pool at McCarran Park. Today there was only Gerald and another girl named Carmen. Carmen was shy, but as I tried to start a conversation Gerald followed me on his bike with his pea shooter. I heard the ping, ping, as he got off his bike and aimed the pea shooter at me. He connected a few times and the hard peas landed on my head and once near my face. It hurt and I begged him to stop but he just laughed and chased me home on his bike. I was safe, I thought as I closed the iron project door designed to keep out all Gerald's.

That night I woke up in a cold sweat, feeling a lump in my throat. I panicked when I swallowed and felt an obstruction. Like the Princess and the Pea. I could not sleep that whole night, I was dying because of Gerald... I tossed and turned and the next morning I would not go to school.

"Gerald shot a pea and it's stuck in my throat," I said to my mother.

"Go to school."

I started crying and holding my throat. I knew the pea was in there. I would die of asphyxiation. My mother understood desperation. She walked me to Saint Catherine's hospital, a dusty old building destined for demolition. I sat in an almost empty emergency room until an ancient nun walked in. She listened to my hysterical story with the "crazy eyes" look I would get to know too well.

She peered down my throat with a flashlight squinting for a while and said, "There's nothing in there," so we walked home.

I felt that pea in my throat for a week, but unlike the princess, the certainty of the pea did not announce my royalty. It announced the arrival of panic and like Rapunzel, I longed to let down my golden hair and be released from my prison of fear.

CHAPTER 11

YOUR'E NOT THE BOSS OF ME

August 24, 1964, was my fourteenth birthday and the day depression and anxiety announced its arrival and intention to stay around awhile. It started with a lecture from my mother about how bad I had become since turning twelve. "Hoodlum" she shouts.

I promised to change and she gave me five dollars and told me not to spend it. I immediately went to the bookstore and bought the "Carpetbaggers", a book that was supposed to be sexy. After that, I was hit up by Maurice, my friend Renee's scary brother, who bullied me into lending him a dollar of my birthday booty. I knew I would never get paid back, but he was so aggressive it scared me.

I went to the candy store and bought an orange drink and a bag of potato chips and ate them on the project bench. My friends were all at the McCarran Park Pool, where I was forbidden to go alone, and since my mother never went out. I was stuck in the steamy projects feeling sad. I found some comfort in being able to eat food I chose, and went back to the apartment. My mother told me she would teach me how to iron. She had a weird look in her eyes as she set up the ironing board. She rambled on how she did all the work and I was a lazy slob. I had learned to shut her out, but I remember that hot August afternoon, holding that heavy hot iron, sweating, listening to her rant on how I was older now and had to return to the good girl I had once been. I really wanted her to accept me so I promised to be better, but as she droned on, I felt a wave of depression hit me, a tsunami I would get to know well.

The Carpetbagger's proved as salacious as promised and as soon as my mother got tired of teaching me the intricacies of ironing, I escaped to my room to read the whole novel and then the good parts over and over. I had become obsessed with sex since I discovered boys and orgasms.

I couldn't stay as good as she wanted for long and started to answer her back when she wanted a piece of me.

"Leave me alone," though mild, irritated her to no end. For me, being free and alone is part of what my agoraphobia is about. I just wanted to be my own person and keep my secrets no matter how bad I felt about them.

That same year, my mother would find my diary and read about my how my boyfriend of two months asked me to jerk him off. I felt betrayed when she called me a tramp and predicted my life as a streetwalker was imminent.

My own words had betrayed me. The boy, Donnie, never liked me much. We only hung out because Ana, my best friend was going out with my classmate Gabe, a boy she would end up marrying. Donnie was Gabe's best friend. I wrote how he taught me how to please him with my hands and how he came in my long blonde hair. My mother had found my secret hiding place under my bed, broke the flimsy lock and read all this and also how humiliated I felt afterwards trying to wash out the unfamiliar substance from my hair.

My mother's prediction that no boy would like me also proved untrue. Yes, I had a bad acne condition, didn't wear the latest styles, but I had a body that by any measure was hot. In my project world, that meant the curvy ass that Latin boys craved. And my appetite for sex (or the hope of it) was driving me to outsmart my mother.

My mother became more obsessed with me as I became more outspoken. She wanted to know and control every detail and aspect of my life. Yet, if I did something unusual or special she wouldn't mention it. I think she was jealous of the power that youth brings. She became especially interested in my choice of friends. Her sharp tongue tore the project rejects, she said I dragged home to pieces.

Chuchie was a smart girl who wore a patch because of her many eye operations. I was eight and she was twelve when I brought her home and we became very close. She was intelligent and kind but rejected because she was not quite black and didn't speak Spanish though she was. Her mother was Puerto Rican and petite with an accent. Her father was a Black Venezuelan who lived in Harlem with his new wife Ramona. Hilda had many husbands and baby daddy's yet demanded Chuchie's absolute obedience.

Once she charged into Chuchie's room, asking if she was "masturpainting" but Chuchie was secretly smoking outside the window. We cracked up for hours about that. Her mother was as scary as mine was, so we had a lot in common. In fact, my first boyfriend was Danny, her brother, who was a "fairy" according to my mother.

"He spends more time in the mirror than you do and the Jewish ladies on the bench are saying you are dating a "Black fairy" my mother said.

But fairy or not, she was concerned enough to send me away for the summer. I never found out until later that Danny was gay.

I was thirteen and in the eighth grade when Chuchie delivered a letter to me with this sentence. "I am sending you this impromptu epistle to request that you be my queen."

I threw up.

I couldn't believe that this boy who most of the project girls desired wanted me. Add that with words I had to look up in the dictionary and I was delirious but anxious. I was the innocent decoy who hid his, in the closet gay life, but I think he cared for me. We only made out twice in a year, but I never forgot Danny, the first boy I loved.

Chuchie was pronounced crazy by mother. Ana just used me and Rosa was a tramp. She especially was resentful of Ana because she said I jumped whenever Ana beckoned her finger. I was an only child and lonely and grateful for any friendship. Ana was a good friend. She was just shy and we remain close. But when Ana got married and I was the Maid of Honor, my mother said I spent more money and effort on her than on my own wedding.

One day during this time a man with a black suitcase showed up at my house telling me I had to take a blood test because a boy had reported to the authorities that I had sex with him and he had a 'social disease'.

"I'm a virgin," I cried and protested to no avail.

I was so afraid of the blood test I peed my pants, but my mother remained stoic.

I begged, "Please don't do this, I'm innocent."

He took out the scary looking needles and I passed out.

When I woke up, the needle was in my arm and he barked, "Don't move; I've spent enough time with this nonsense already."

I didn't move and the ordeal was over. I crept in my room wracking my brain over who the person might be who falsely accused me of having sex and dirty sex at that. I only thought of Rafael, who was gay and angry because I had been Danny's first girlfriend before him. He had also set me up for his friends to beat me up.

Recently, my sex abuse therapist scared me to the bone, when she suggested it was my mother who called the authorities.

At first I couldn't wrap my mind around this but recalling my mother's look of determination makes this a horrible possibility.

"Hey mom, I was innocent. You know I was."
"Don't look at me like that. Help me and tell this scary man to go away."

"Why are you so quiet and standing still with your hands on your hips?"
Could her mental illness have convinced her I wasn't a virgin but a syphilis carrying whore?
I only know I have an aversion to ironing.

CHAPTER 12

I BECOME TINY

I never thought I would join a gang but in the fall of my ninth year at William J Gaynor Junior High school, I unwittingly became a Lady Horseman. The Horsemen were a gang that ruled my neighborhood. Their enemies were the "Young Saints" a rival gang whose turf was most of South Williamsburg. Though I had heard their names, I never thought I would be involved with them until the unlucky day I decided to play hooky at Rafael's house.

Rafael was part of the group I hung out with and was a very flamboyant gay teenager. Since gay was not a word we used let alone understood, he fooled us by going steady with every girl from our group. I even went out with him for a few days like most of my friends, but he always found a reason to break up with us and still keep us as friends. When he invited us to a gig, (a party arranged during school when your parents were working- also called a set) we went and found ourselves surrounded by friends of his from "El Barrio (Spanish Harlem), where he conducted his secret life. The girls were cold and tough and ignored me Donna, and Ana. I didn't know this party would lead to yet another drama that would add to my anxiety.

I had the lead in the school play. I was Anna in the "King and I", and rehearsed every day after school. My co-star was Roberto Ruiz; a cute boy who didn't know I existed. I had tried out for every play since 7th grade and only now, had proven to Mr. Nelson, our talent teacher, that I had the voice and the personality to pull this off.

Mr. Nelson, a homosexual Black teacher who suffered many indignities from the students, was very talented, played the piano and sang. The other kids called him "faggot" behind his back but I thought that meant he walked with a sway to his hips and used a lot of hand gestures when he spoke, not a bad thing to me.

I worshipped him because he taught me the folk music and Negro spirituals that made me cry with happiness.

If you had decent grades and showed an interest in any artistic endeavor, you were allowed to be in his class for two periods a day. He taught us songs like "Black is the color of my true loves hair", and "I wonder as I wander."

I was not his favorite student since my looks and personality did not shout star to him. But at the final play of my final year at JHS 49, I gave my all at audition. For once, I forgot myself and lifted my alto soprano voice to sweetly hit the high notes with the passion I was always afraid of. He looked at me with surprise; as did the other "talent" students who had laughed at me when I messed up at an audition the previous year. He decided to give me the co- lead along with Norma Estes, a perfect looking girl with half the voice I had but so much body, that a seamstress had to sew me in the ball gown we would share. She would perform on Thursday and Saturday, and I would be Anna on Tuesday and Friday

Norma was his pet, and even though I was the better singer, I knew If I screwed up, I would lose my tenuous grip on fame.

The next day after the party, I was at rehearsal and a virtual army of girls and boys from Harlem were waiting for me outside. I was on stage, and a brave thugette, grabbed a coat from my seat. The coat wasn't mine, and the petite Chinese girl who played Tumptim, screamed and ran after her coat. Mr. Nelson was not amused. I was in a state of panic and could not move from my spot onstage.

Roberto, my king whispered to me. "I'm the leader of the Horsemen; I'll send Lady Cocaine, your friend to help you. I did not know any Lady Cocaine but I was more than grateful because I was quivering and about to faint.

A few minutes later, my oldest friends Rosalinda, Chuchie, and Gloria walked in. Gloria was "Lady Cocaine." I didn't even know they were Lady Horsemen. They were both tall and tough and loved me. I breathed a sigh of relief as they were followed by an opposing army behind them, led by an unusual, to say the least, boy who looked almost exactly like Alfred E. Neumann from "Mad Magazine", or the Latino version with red hair, freckles, and a husky physique. He was called Lobo, (wolf) in Spanish and after the ruckus he whispered to me that now, since they saved me I would not only have to join the gang but be his woman. Ay, Ay, Ay, as my father would say.

I found out later, my friend Donna got beat up and her glasses smashed, and although they looked for Ana, she had friends and brothers who backed her up. I told Ana my dilemma and she reluctantly said she would also join the gang to keep me company. I, however, had to walk through the apache line, which is literally getting kicked in a gang.

When I walked to the park, I felt I was walking the final mile. I tried to remember the first song I sang in the "King and I".

"Whenever I feel afraid I hold my head up high and whistle a happy tune and no one ever knows I'm afraid."

Needless to say it didn't work.

When I arrived a line of girls and guys had formed and I would have to enter through the middle. They waited for me and my pounding heart told me the gig was up.

I can't explain the reasons I walked through that line but when I did, I lost my fear. I'm always afraid of things that probably won't happen, but in real danger I am dead calm.

I am small and the members didn't want to kill me, I hoped, but I walked through the punches and kicks as fast as my short legs could carry me.

When I exited the line, Lobo was standing proudly and smiled and said, "You are in the gang. Your name is Tiny because you're a tiny terror."

As I looked at my friend's shocked face, I couldn't help but feel proud of myself for facing the fear with only a few bruises. I went home and ran into the bathroom and locked the door. I was a bit black and blue at dinner but my mother looked at me in silence. My mother's mantra was, "Don't tell me anything bad," and this was bad.

Lobo told me Ana didn't have to be jumped in because she spoke Spanish. She said she would never have done it anyway.

I hung out with the gang between rehearsals for my play and managed to keep my double life a secret for a time. I once was asked to carry weapons for the rumble with the Saints. I didn't hesitate because I felt I belonged to something and was important to them and feeling important to someone felt special. Even playing the lead in "The king and I," didn't make me feel that way.

At the last minute, my mother refused to let me out of the house. I felt so ashamed the next day, but they were benign about my situation and just said I missed out on a good rumble.

I did start to stay home from school and drink T -bird wine with Lobo. He was surprisingly respectful and we would lie down together clothed and make out. Sometimes Ana, (gang name Chica) hung out with us. She liked a boy named JR, who had a cape like Zorro, all the Puerto Rican project boys' hero. I would come home with my lips stained red from cheap wine and go to bed after making believe I was eating my dinner.

One early evening, the doorbell rang and rang. It was my father's day with us and he opened the door to see Lobo, Shadow and JR at my door with somber faces. He jumped back at the sight and shut the door in their faces, saying they had the wrong door. The next day, my mother opened the door to Gypsy, a scrawny light skinned girl a few years older than me. She asked my mother, "Do you have a daughter with a blonde ponytail and pimples?"

"Nice description", my mother said. Gypsy was led into the living room carrying a baby in a blue blanket, my mother uncommonly hospitable.

"Your daughter is sleeping with my husband, my baby's father."

She pointed to the bundle in her arms like we didn't know what a baby was. Now, that got my mothers attention. She had always thought I was boy crazy and this was her proof. I had gotten close to Lobo but he never tried to get into my unmentionables. I liked him, maybe loved him because he protected me and said he cared about me and though he was like a cartoon character, he was mine or so I thought.

"No, No," I said, as they both looked at me with doubt.

I didn't know he was married. "I didn't, I won't see him again, I promise." Mommy didn't mention he had been in our living room alone with me while she was locked in her room reading.

The next day I was summoned for a meeting with "Blue Moon". I had never met her but knew this menacing woman/girl towering over me was the leader of the Lady Horsemen.

"I hear you've disrespected Gypsy by flaunting your relationship with Lobo. The gang saw you at the movies kissing him."

I tried to defend myself but she stopped me with a slap. She kept on slapping me until it felt my head would fall off.

If you want to stay in the gang or alive you can't see him again, she repeated, "You do want to stay in don't you?"

"Yes, Yes", I lied. And, with a final slap, she allowed me to leave.

I walked home, and could not speak when my mother said anything. She never mentioned my red cheeks, the blood trickling down my face or the fact I wouldn't leave my room for dinner. That night I went to the kitchen and took a sharp knife from the kitchen drawer. I wanted to die, but instead, I cut my arm in little vertical lines of blood. I found out that the cutting calmed me and as the tears finally fell, I killed Tiny.

Leaving the gang was as easy as stepping on a project cockroach. They didn't really like me or need me as much as I had thought. I wasn't even missed. I didn't go to school for a few days, and went back to my old life of school and rehearsals running home like a terrified jackrabbit.

The night the play opened, Roberto never mentioned Lobo, Gypsy, or Blue Moon. And when we waltzed around the stage in "Shall we dance," I was floating, enraptured, as I forgot myself and the real life drama I was in, and became Anna and really, really believed I was in Siam.

At graduation, I came back to life as Mr. Nelson who never forgot the neighborhood drama, gave Norma numerous awards for her role in the play and for being the "all around talent" student. I got *nada*. I looked down in shame and depression with the knowledge I was a big nothing and I had messed up as usual.

Even though I received an invitation from the "High School of Performing Arts" to attend their audition, and I was told I was so talented, Tiny refused to die and I continued to cut.

CHAPTER 13

BETRAYAL AT HORSESHIT BEACH

In the summer just before I turned fifteen, I stayed with my brother for a week. I rarely did this because the Bronx was my mother's least favorite borough of New York City. Nestor was my favorite half brother and inherited my father's magnetic appeal to such a degree that even my mother admired him. He shared that when he and his brother arrived from Puerto Rico, my mother refused to take them in until our grandmother arrived in New York to care for them, and they had to stay in a foster home for a while. I vaguely remember my father pushing my mother against the wall when she called them the "N" word. Nestor said it was because his brother Angel was dark and she was ashamed. Nestor eventually won her over and Angel, the youngest son ended up living with my parents when he became sick and homeless.

I used to have severely painful periods in my early teens and the first part of the week I spent was in a haze of pain. The first day of my period I sat white faced in their rocking chair praying it would not move. The pain was so intense I couldn't speak or move a muscle, even with two Midol's, a girl's best friend for that time of the month.

The next day, my brother persuaded me to go to their friend's house on the train and I remember hanging on the pole so hard, my knuckles turned white. I got dizzy and my brother had to carry me down the subway stairs. That part was nice, even in my delirium, I remember that. The third day was always better when the flow began, and I mean flow. I was then afraid to stain everything in sight but didn't feel the pain anymore. That weekend, the ending of my period, the family went to the beach, "Orchard Beach" or as my mother called it "Horseshit Beach."

I was happy that day. I wore my first bikini and I looked as inviting as a young girl with a hot figure could be. My bikini had yellow polka dots and my brother sang. "She's afraid to go out of the water; she wore an itsy bitsy teeny weenie yellow polka dot bikini." I loved when he teased me and proud that he thought I was pretty.

Who should we see when we entered the picnic area, but my father with a dark haired plump youngish woman and a child sitting on a blanket? Before I could think, my father ran up to me obviously as surprised to see me there as I was shocked to see him.

"I have a lady friend with me", he told me with a nervous look in his eyes. "Don't say anything about this to your mother."

I looked again. The dark haired woman had breasts like two watermelons and gave me a sullen look I would get to know better in the future as she glared at me with stupid eyes. I didn't know how to respond. I really believed my father was home with his sick mother all the time he wasn't at our home, which was most of the time. I didn't see a sign of my grandmother at Horseshit Beach.

But standing in front of me stood a young girl with braids, braces, and a big smile. She ran up to me.

"I'm your sister Carol."

If icicles had a tone, it would have been warmer as I slowly said, "I don't have a sister. I'm an only child."

Her happy smile faded as I ran away with tears streaming from my eyes.

My brother Nestor ran after me. "Baby, I'm sorry you had to find out like this, but Wilma has been with daddy since she was eighteen, and she's his other wife."

"Other wife, I said, what is that?"

I ran away thinking that little girl has what I always longed for, my father's time and attention. All I had of my father, which wasn't much, was at that moment, stripped away from me by this happy girl. She was at the beach with my father and his other wife, while I was abandoned to my crazy mother who never went out.

"No, No," I said aloud while a couple looked up from their open mouthed kiss. I had held on to my tenuous title as daddy's only girl, and even though I only saw him a few times a week, he couldn't be cheating on me with this "Carol."

I ran through the sand, feeling my long hair swing in the light breeze. Not thinking, I ran into the ocean feeling it slow my racing heart. A cute boy with brown eyes approached me speaking broken English and we started chatting with the few Spanish words I knew and he beckoned me to go deeper in the water.

"I can't swim."

"Don't worry. I'll take care of you."

Feeling reckless, I let him cradle me in his arms as he walked in the ocean. He never touched my body or spoke at first, but spun around slowly and I felt the pain drain from my body by the flow of the ocean. Then he kissed me tenderly. I spent the rest of the afternoon clinging to this strange boy who told me his name was Oswaldo Pepper. I laughed at the odd name. He was from Ecuador, and he called me his blonde mermaid. I gave him my phone number as I saw my brother frantically calling me to join the "family party," but I wouldn't speak to my father. I learned that day that boys and romance were better medications for pain than Midol or aspirin.

Oswaldo Pepper, the boy at the beach, became the first boy who proposed to me and I broke his heart when I fell for his"Casanova" friend Gustavo, who dumped me when I wouldn't have sex with him. All I remember of Oswaldo now, is that he called me silently and played

records in a mixture of Spanish and his native Quechan Indian dialect.
“You never loved me, and you betrayed me.” I felt his pain, but I wasn’t destined to become Mrs. Pepper.
I was also betrayed by my first love; my elusive father that summer day at “Horseshit beach, and like my menstrual cramps, pain is pain.

Jan 9th

It is only 4 o'clock. I am very sick. Marilyn called, Ray called. Please let me be quiet for the rest of the day. I don't want to upset Carl. He wanted to stay at the little ladies house. But when he called, I acted sick and he came home. Please don't let me upset him. I don't want to act up. Please God let me be quiet. I want to act normal. I was very sick all day. Please God let me act normal. Give me a little peace and I will. She made supper for him. I am so sorry I am so sick. I want hope so desperately. He couldn't even stay. When I got home from the hospital, I was sick but now I'm terrible. I need help. But where? It is 6:30. I want to watch TV. God help me. I feel so sick, let me hang on. Benny our neighbor is in the house. I hope I will be Ok till 9 o'clock time for my pills. Benny called the police about Angie being missing for 3 days. The police say they can't list him as a missing person because he is 47 years old. I think he is dead. Carl is very upset. But I think he is better off dead. He has diabetes and cancer of the liver. He has been eating large quantities of sweets. He was practically in a coma when he left. I don't think he should have stayed here. In fact both of us should have remained in the hospital.

PART 3

TROUBLE

'INSANITY DESTROYS REASON BUT NOT WIT"

NATHANIEL EMMONS
AMERICAN THEOLIGIAN 1745-1840

CHAPTER 14

THE VIRGIN DRAMA QUEEN

My mom and I both got slapped on our respective wedding days. My Jewish mother was thirty- five and got slapped by her youngest brother Morty who called her a whore for marrying my father, a Puerto Rican. I was sixteen and bitch slapped by a dwarf. Now, they are called little people but Susan was only little in size. I had missed dress rehearsal for our opening night of our first big gig at the Hanson Theatre in Brooklyn. We were the Williamsburg Players and I was one of the main players. We were performing "Bits and Pieces." Jeffrey James, our choreographer's creation. Susan was the general manager and piano player and took our big break seriously. Seriously, so did I, but after our wedding ceremony at my uncle Pejean's house in the Bronx, Jose, my new husband and his loser cousin Juan got us lost in his beater car. I showed up a few minutes before show time with a headache from trying to understand my vows. The pastor was my uncle's friend and I had to answer "si" in the right place and my Spanish was more "no" at the time. I should have said no.

Jose Rivera was a simple man from Puerto Rico and even though I said I would never marry a Jibaro (hillbilly fresh off the boat) he had the necessary qualifications- a job and a willingness to marry me and take me out of hell. He never had a proper father. He was brought up by his grandmother with his real mother living next door with her husband and a slew of children. Until he was seventeen, he thought his mother was his aunt. Dona Lola was tough as nails with a sense of humor as dry as an exceptionally dry martini.

My mother, at first threatened me with marriage because she thought I had lost my virginity when I stayed out all night with him. She later changed her mind when I looked too happy about it, and so it was arranged over her "dead body." She wouldn't listen that I was a virgin. But she wouldn't sign the papers so my father signed. Maybe he knew I had to get away so I got married without the blessing or attendance of my mother.

The night we had supposedly done "it", we slept in his small furnished room in Dean Street in Brooklyn. He was lonely and adored me. I remember one thing that touched me. On his dresser sat a bottle of Hask hair dressing. He said he was told he looked like Elvis and used this product to puff his hair up. We were both alone so I undressed and we slept curled in each others arms.

I was a technical virgin for two years. I could not open my legs so the marriage wasn't consummated. I wanted a child as many lonely girls do. I thought that would be the answer to all my problems. I just wanted to love something. In those days if you were married you had to leave school, in case you would corrupt the other girls talking about your sex life. My sex life was the same foreplay Jose and I did before we married, but I left school with a strange excitement of not having to go anywhere.

Then, I had the bright idea to go to a famous fertility specialist, a husband and wife team I had read about in a book. I paid twenty five dollars for a consultation. That was a fortune for a poor young couple starting out, but I have never let money deter me from getting what I wanted and I wanted a baby. When they tried to examine me, I became hysterical. The woman doctor tried first. My legs were frozen shut.

"You don't need fertility treatments, she said, you need to open you legs and have sex first." Then we will see if you get pregnant." Then the husband tried, failed and said,

"You need a therapist."

I didn't agree and went to a medical doctor to rupture my hymen. I went through an ordeal called a hymenectomy with general anesthesia. I remember the nurse shaving my pubic area with me jumping all over the table.

"If you can't handle this honey, don't even think about having a baby," she said. I woke up to a tube attached to my bladder and realized I had made a bad decision. The woman in the next bed was thirty- nine and had hemorrhoids so painful they had to be operated on. She wanted to change places with me.

To make matters worse, I was given a lecture on proper hygiene when a nurse or hemorrhoid woman said I smelled down there. Even then, I was flabbergasted at that indignity. I had tubes in me and couldn't pee when they removed them. A kind head nurse turned on the water and stayed until I peed. I never forgot that kindness but it was ruined by this person lecturing me on how to wash myself. I was seventeen and meek but anger bubbled inside of me and I was so full of anger that if I had known my inner child then, she would be Stephen King's Carrie. To make matters worse, Joe kept complaining that the doctor popped my cherry and I should marry him.

But on my wedding day, I sang "I feel pretty" and "Somewhere" from West Side Story, I began to panic as I felt less than pretty and the "Somewhere" I wanted to be was home. Usually on the stage, I could forget myself and be in the character or song, but, I began to remember Susan's screwed up face when she swung at me. It was anything but pretty, and my cheeks burned and stung. I focused instead on my new husband Jose in the audience beaming at me with pride and by the time my finale "Tonight" started I had lost myself in the joy of performing. I was officially a newlywed at sixteen and free from my mother's iron rule and insanity (or so I thought).

It's not a contradiction to have an anxiety disorder and be a performer. It was a distraction for me like eating, reading and dancing. I forgot myself and was able to feel free to be somewhere and someone else. I am good at being someone else.

I was never told I had talent in singing but I loved it so much that I tried with my one powerful resource, my mother, to sing as much as possible in front of any audience my mother could bribe, beg or threaten. She was good at threatening. When I was ten year old she pestered the Williamsburg Community Center for a rent free venue and with the promise of the five dollars worth of candy she bought, I drew a crowd as big as any rock stars.

I felt a sense of power while I sang rock and roll tunes like the "Shirelles Will you still love me tomorrow." I used my falsetto to sing Peggy March's "I will follow him." I even talked my friends into being in the show. Donna, my friend from my building danced the Irish jig, and my best friend Chuchie sang like an angel. I was never jealous. I was proud. I had the candy. I never felt as confident as when I faced that crowd. I never panicked and though my mother never praised me, she was supportive of my endeavor. I don't know why she turned against me when I began to succeed.

I never imagined I had talent for singing or anything else until one day at Camp Vacamas
sleep away camp in New Jersey; I won a contest I never intended to enter. I was outside the audition room with a retarded girl who always said "I wonder" after every sentence. One example was "I wonder if we're going swimming, I wonder." Naturally she hooked on to the other untouchable in the bunk, me. We were pretending to be holding our own contest and I was singing "Summertime" in a soprano falsetto register. Suddenly

a counselor came running out. "Who was that singing?" she asked.

She looked at me strangely when I tentatively raised my hand. I was the girl with the dirty face and hands who other campers avoided. I was the scaredy cat, the girl who couldn't and wouldn't learn how to swim and cried when we were forced to row on the lake because I was scared of the boat tipping over. No one picked me for any teams, and when I was standing there last, the captain would inevitably say, "Oh no, not her." It reminded me of kindergarten when we were dancing to "The farmer in the dell", and I asked my mother why I was always the cheese that stood alone. She was not amused.

But that day, I was a winner. I wasn't that unpopular girl with poor hygiene who couldn't cope with self care on my own.

When I sang, I was powerful. I was the girl with the big voice. My self confidence grew and I literally found a voice and friends at camp, not the popular in crowd, but not only the "rejected." Being memorable for talent became my reason for breathing.

My cousin Cindy went to the same camp and I worshipped her. She was popular and sweet. I was so proud to own her as my kin. She stuck up for me when I was teased and I could talk to her. I remember her big brown eyes always listening while we laughed and were normal together. One night in the bunk, she started crying because she was homesick, and the counselor came over to hug her. I felt so sad, I started crying too. I said I was homesick too and though my crying was real, it was not for the same reason. I cried for the life that Cindy was crying for. Her loving, normal parents, who doted on her and let her stay up until nine at night, when I had to go to bed early like a baby; her parents who didn't scream, even when she decided to cut her hair at five and become an Indian with a beaded headband.. I cried for a hug, that I didn't get at home since I was six. I cried with such passion and noticed the counselor wasn't as effusive with my hug and seemed to come over to my bunk a bit reluctantly but I took what I could get. I always do. My acting career had begun.

My dream of being noticed started at Radio City Music Hall. My mother was obsessed with movies and every time the movie changed we took the trek to Manhattan. I got dressed up and sometimes my Cindy slept over the night before.

We always went on Saturday mornings when the price was lower, and I remember waiting as the usher led us in to wait at the closed door in front of the seat entrance. Dimmed lights, red patterned carpet and a huge chandelier greeted us. To the left was a huge staircase that represented all that was classy to me. We were then led to our plush red seats and I remember the excited yet respectful hum of the audience I would later become addicted to. Then in the lower left side of the huge stage, an organist would rise from the pit and played music I was unfamiliar with. Yet, I somehow I knew I was in a kind of a church and never wanting to stop praying there.

I was mesmerized by "Gigi", whisked away to Hong Kong, with the "Wonderful world of Suzi Wong" and laughed myself silly at Doris Day's "Please don't eat the daises."

At the end of the movie, my eyes blinked, as the light and the buzz signaled the Rockettes to take over. I would always cry at the end when their famous high kicks ended. I couldn't believe there were woman so confident, beautiful and talented, ok, and tall. Yet, the best part, was about to begin. We joined the throngs going downstairs to the luxury of the restroom. Downstairs, elegance I only saw on the screen awaited me. I always peeked at the painting (Men without Women) by Stuart Davis in the gentleman's lounge. I remember this painting as a modern even cartoonish depiction of men's toys, playing cards autos, boats, yet even my young eyes spotted the outline of a woman's figure in the mix. There were also sculpture and statuary worthy of Rome, combined with the art deco of a Fred Astaire picture. The powder room shouted elegance with individual cubicles, each with a mirror where I would imagine putting on make up and leaping on the stage. I knew then my life in the projects with my parents was not the life I was meant to have and would willingly have stayed there if asked.

After the show we ate lunch at a Chinese restaurant a few notches above in quality than the one we always went to in Brooklyn. As we ate fried rice, my cousin and I opened our fortune cookies and toasted our futures clicking our water glasses in unison. Daydreaming, my favorite pastime took over and I saw myself clearly; a star on stage and could even hear the clapping in my head as I took a bow. But when I was entered into that singing contest and won, I felt normal and ready for stardom.

On my wedding day on that other stage, I knew I had arrived. I was free and talented. I would be famous despite the slap. I didn't know then that life and mental illness would have other plans for me.

CHAPTER 15

Honeymoon in Puerto Rico

A year after our marriage Jose and I went on a delayed honeymoon to Puerto Rico. I was working as a temp for "Manpower" for the "United Jewish Appeal of Greater New York" as a clerk. I saved every penny and we went on my, then, dream trip to Puerto Rico where my father was born. We had our brand of strange sex under the "mosquitera" (large netting) over the wooden bed with a photo of a very Spanish looking Jesus. This was my first trip outside of The New York City Tri State Area, and I was excited and nervous.

Jose Luis or Joe as I called him had been raised by his grandmother. When he found out, his aunt next door was his real mother; he left Puerto Rico at eighteen but still loved his grandmother and wrote to her ever faithfully, every week. Dona Lola was his rock, his only form of stability until he met me. His loneliness is what attracted me to him. I felt a connection with the young lost soul he was then. He would always start his letter with, "I hope this letter finds you and the family in the best of health." I learned a bit of Spanish by reading his letters with him. They seemed very boring to me, and our life was anything but that, but I knew what it was to lie about your life.

We arrived in San Juan on a steamy June day. I made my first faux pas by mistaking his mother for his grandmother. She was not amused but to my seventeen year old mind, she looked way older than thirty six. Hell, to my sixty year old minds eye she looks ancient. When I was seventeen- twenty was old to me. We proceeded to rent a car and driver to the Eastern mountain town of Comerio, not far from the town of Caguas where my father was born and my grandfather Isidro Mendoza lived with his wife who was not my grandmother.

As the car meandered around the mountain in smaller and smaller circles, I had to stop the car and vomit. The combination of my first plane trip on Eastern Airlines, the bumpy road straight up a mountain and my anxiety at meeting his family had reached its limit. Joe and the driver laughed as I emptied my guts and we finally got to their sleepy Puerto Rican mountain town.

In the center of Comerio, there was a lovely town square and a few restaurants and shops. But we were entering "Bda Pasarell" across a bridge, the poor part of town. We arrived at two houses next to each other which would be called a hovel if the observer was generous. They were like boxes with no indoor plumbing at all. Outside was a cold shower and I mean mountain cold and next to that a smelly latrine I would come to know as the monster. The "Latrina" needed a ladder to climb up to the seat. It didn't have one. The smell was so powerful and noxious; I could only describe it as hellish.

The whole family which included his real mother's seven kids, her new husband and various onlookers, stood outside to watch the white fake Puerto Rican blonde. They all wore huge smiles but I didn't see the grandmother and asked for her politely. No one spoke English, so I had to have everything translated by Joe. Inside one of the houses was his grandmother at the stove cooking. Now, Joe had always told me to look up when I saw his grandmother because she was so tall. He told me this a lot especially before the trip so I looked up and didn't see anyone. I had to look lower and lower and finally a woman who was barely four feet four stared up at me from her stove. I wanted to laugh. I tried not to laugh. Ok, I laughed. I laughed and laughed and had to be helped to a chair.

"Is she normal?" his grandmother asked in Spanish to Joe, but Joe was laughing too.

"So you're here," she said dryly.

She was as witty as a leprechaun on pot yet tough as her Taino Indian ancestors and I tried to redeem myself by hugging her. She let herself be hugged but wasn't buying what this young blonde teenager was selling.

In the living room, was a huge television and I thought it was strange not to have indoor plumbing or water, yet have such a deluxe living room with the standard Latino picture of the last supper and the twin pink peacocks on the wall. The dinner was delicious and I knew it was pig's feet because it looked like pigs feet.

"This meat is delicious. What is it?"

"Special Comerio pork", one of his rascally brothers said. I played along to make them laugh,

"Do you know what you just ate?"

"Yes, Comerio special pork."

"No, it's its pig's feet." I pretended to faint and scream. They fell on the floor laughing and I thought I was pretty smart, until I saw the way they washed dishes; in a sink outside the kitchen window with a hose.

There were cows outside that would moo in the morning and "Coqui" tree frogs that would chirp all night, yet I never slept more soundly. In the morning, as the grandmother would make the coffee and toast they all ate for breakfast, I took a shower. This was a time for jubilation for the younger naughty brothers. They gathered to hear me scream as the freezing water hit my body and sometimes peek in the many holes in the flimsy structure and say "Hi."

One day we went on an outing to see my grandfather in Caguas and we brought Joe's oldest sister Milagros, who was eighteen, sweet and had clear caramel skin and flowing black hair. After our visit which was brief and cold, I had the feeling my grandfather was as interested in knowing me as my father was. He looked like an older version of my father with blue eyes and white hair and his wife stiffly poured us lemonade. One thing my grandfather was interested in was Milagros. He kept saying what a beautiful girl she was. I felt left out, unpretty and worthless as usual and became very depressed on the way home.

Joe cheered me up saying with his Puerto Rican fatalism, "You can't change him. Your father told me he left your grandmother and the only two of his kids who survived, your dad and Pejean almost starved after they broke up. Look he has a damn cigar factory and your father had nada."

I wanted to be the object of my grandfather's attention as he had only seen me once before and I also wanted to be pretty and slim. I was already dealing with my weight obsession and weighed 130 pounds when arriving and was called plump. If only I could get down to Milagros size, I would be acceptable. It was my grandfather's lust for dark women that made him pay attention to Milagros, not my weight, but I kept on thinking 117 pounds like Milagros. I have to get to that weight somehow.

Going to the "Latrina" proved to be too hard - literally. I was keeping it in until we got to a real bathroom and became constipated even with all the beans I was eating. Finally, Dona Lola gave me "La escupidera" a basin to defecate in. One afternoon after Joe and I returned from sightseeing, his whole family stood outside laughing and speaking Spanish to Joe. Again, I saw no trace of Dona Lola, but got an earful of Spanish directed to me when I entered her kitchen. I had not emptied the basin in the Latrine and delectable odors had been filling her kitchen.

She yelled,"Empty your own shit into the Latrine before you leave and don't hide it under your bed like a present!"

I was ashamed and pretended not to understand Spanish yet I detected a sense of fun in her.

Oh, the family loved to see the stupid fake Puerto Rican make mistake after mistake. They teased yet I never felt meanness in their teasing but for a seventeen year old virgin, shit is humiliating.

In the evenings, the whole town would congregate outside and drink beer and my husband was no exception. He wanted me to stay in a strange tiny house with his young brothers while he gallivanted with his look-alike cousin Tony. I hated Tony, because of his arrogance. He lived in the center of town and his mother owned a restaurant and he hated me. How dare his poor cousin have a blonde wife? He urged my husband to hang out with their friends in the square in the evening and leave me in that hovel alone. I got angrier and angrier and one of his brothers motioned me to follow him to the square where I saw Tony and Joe flirting and drinking with two young girls.

I faced him and said "goodbye" and marched back to the room where I started packing. He came back, not right away and I told him I would meet him in San Juan, where we were planning to go in two days. He convinced me to stay the few remaining days and he would act right. He explained in Puerto Rico, men just hung with their friends, and nothing was going on. I relented as always.

Now, all week I had been asking for a bar of soap as I had forgotten to bring one. I would meekly walk up to Dona Lola and ask her in English for soap but never got it. The last evening, she called me into the kitchen and in front of Joe, said with fake disgust in Spanish.

"Tell her I cooked her soup all day so she better eat it."

Joe started laughing and told me in Spanish "sopa" is soup and she thought I was asking for soup. "Jabon" means soap. I ate the soup, "Asapao" one of Puerto Rico's National dishes, delicious soupy rice with chicken. The next morning I said goodbye to my new family and when I hugged Dona Lola she hugged me back. I was so touched; I got warm all over and didn't want to leave.

The last night I got pregnant under the "mosquitera." Somehow Jose's sperm made that big leap. It must have been a super determined sperm because I stayed a technical virgin for many years even after the virgin birth of my daughter. So tight were my muscles, that my daughter's birth on July 29, 1969 was named by hospital "Delivery on the moon." My mind was determined... No one would get inside my insides.

CHAPTER 16

WHICH WITCH?

Agoraphobia means fear of the marketplace. At seventeen, the marketplace was one of the only places I was not afraid of. Oh, I had the classic panic attacks when I was in line with my groceries and without warning, feel I was dying. I had to run out abandon my shopping cart and try to look normal while catching my breath that had left my limp body. But the difference was I always went back. My food addiction fought my panic attacks and most of the time won. I had to get my fix. Pastrami sandwiches, as many as I could stuff down, pounds of potato salad, rolls, coke, potato chips and vanilla ice cream melted and slithered down my throat. As soon as the world stopped spinning, I went back to the store and came home clutching my drugs tightly, my heart still pounding from the panic attack.

I had to eat it all and dispose of all the evidence before my husband Jose came home. That part was hard because after all those carbs, I was fighting the urge to pass out. I managed to wake up in time to also do a bit of cleaning to answer his inevitable question. “What did you do all day?” I was seventeen and already deep into my madness of compulsive overeating and fear, and giddy that my mother couldn’t stop me.

I almost stopped going out at all after believing, I mean really, really believing there was a witch that was following me. The woman showed up wherever I was, and gave me meaningful scary looks. I would get panicky when I saw her and ran away. She had long grey hair and a pointed nose. I began to make excuses to stay home so I wouldn’t see her. If I had to go out, I would run to and fro like a frightened doe, darting my eyes back and forth. I saw her in the back of other woman’s heads, in crowds and in stores. A face would suddenly turn and it was her- I think. In my mind she lived in the cellars that were the storage areas of Brooklyn stores. I was especially afraid of stepping on a cellar lest she pull me in.

I felt safe at home and comfy with my food and "Dark Shadows" a scary soap opera which come to think of it had a witch named Angelique featured in it. I stopped washing or combing my hair. It seemed too tiring and I ran faster and faster to pick up my food, my wild hair flying in the wind. One day I saw the witch, and she startled at the sight of me. It was my own white face reflected in a supermarket mirror. I started to think I was the witch. Had the witch turned me into a witch? Which witch? Was I mad?

I was scared, really scared and the next few years would find me seeking the security of my home until that also became unbearable.

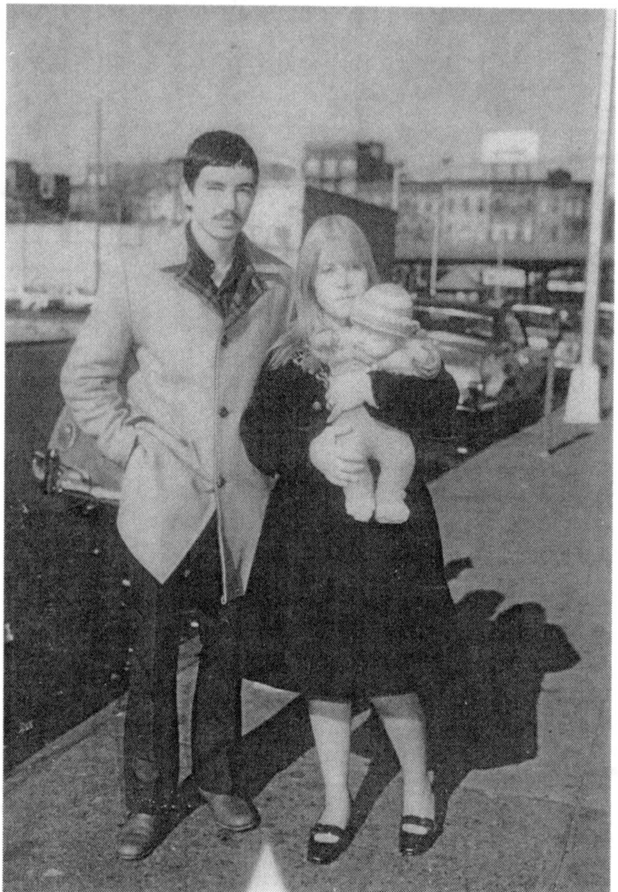

CHAPTER 17

MOTHER MCCREE

I don't know who Mother McCree was, but I suspect she's a cross between Amy Winehouse and the devil. My mother nicknamed me M.M. when I had my first baby at eighteen. I admit it was a bad idea to come straight home from the hospital with my baby to my mother's house but I was young, scared and my mother had insisted. I stayed a week there and found out I was also incompetent, unworthy and plain stupid.

Her expression, "I'm only giving you constructive criticism," didn't help the name calling. The stupid part according to my mother started with naming my daughter Elena. My mother declared she would rename her Ellen because Elena sounded Puerto Rican. Elena is Puerto Rican. I was incompetent because I had never held or diapered a baby and my attempts were not up to my mother's exact standards. She took over the care of my new baby while I looked on like a moronic bystander at my own funeral. I was unworthy because Elena was small, wonderful and beautiful and I didn't deserve to be her mother.

I lasted there a week before running for my life. Mom's shrill, "Mother McCree come here and watch me," combined with post-partum depression recreated my original house of horrors.

Elena must have sensed the discord in the house because she screamed all night and that was the only time my mother wasn't ready to grab her out of her basinet. But I was so tired, I started resenting this strange new person who wouldn't shut up and hating myself for feeling that way.

After I left, my mother as contrary as ever, paid for a housekeeper to come home with me for two weeks. I was so grateful I couldn't stop crying when I entered my studio apartment with my baby, I didn't even care my mother didn't trust my competence to care for my child. I didn't trust it either. After another sleepless night, the downstairs bell rang and an angel in the body of Ella waited patiently for me to open the door.

Ella was an African American woman of substantial weight and heart. Under her care, I slept, the baby slept and my depression lifted like a pink balloon on a calm yet windy day. While she cleaned my house and cooked my lunch, I cared for my baby with an ease that lifted my spirits and raised my self-esteem. My house was peaceful, I was peaceful. Even my hard- working, hard partying husband Jose seemed, at least for a while to want to stay home more and play daddy.

Ella had a spirit that brought lightness and confidence to my panicked heart. We chatted over the tea she introduced to me. Before Ella, I hated tea; but straight without cream and sugar was another story.

She gently lectured me on the one plain hamburger with ketchup I allowed myself to eat per day. I was punishing myself for gaining thirty pounds and being mocked by the labor room nurse. But Ella let me do what I wanted. She taught me how to be a mother and encouraged me to be happy. She had ten children and for two weeks I was her eleventh child. I gave her a carpet sweeper when she left. I watched with amazement as she fixed, cleaned and took it home.

After she left, I began to believe that staying home was the way to keep the peace she brought to my life. I made excuses not to go out. Who would want to leave this bliss I told myself. And I didn't unless I was forced to.

When I went shopping once a week, I put the baby in the stroller and went over to the park. The park had a contingent of mothers with baby carriages who greeted each other warmly. They didn't know me or attempt to invite me in their clique, but I sat there with my GED studying guide content to study while half- listening to the foreign life of a Bensonhurst Italian wife and mother. I wasn't as much jealous of their close family ties as amazed families could be supportive and close. I had gotten booted out of high school when I admitted I was married, I guess the reason being; a married student would influence other girls to have the sex they were already having.

I braced myself to leave the house and took the three day GED test in Manhattan, and surprised myself by receiving the highest score in science, not my best subject. Then, with all my strength, took a baby step and registered for two classes at New York City Community College in Brooklyn: journalism and drama. I remember renting a typewriter for my final paper for journalism class. My topic was the deeper meaning of "Sesame Street", the only subject I could write five pages on at the time. I was severely marked down for not putting footnotes at the bottom of my paper. The stern journalist said to me, "Weren't you listening in class to even the basic principles?" I passed with a D and felt ashamed but the drama class taught method acting and I got an A for acting unhappy and scared. When the "act normal and joyful" part came, I failed miserably.
The non-acting happy part came after class eating potato pancakes with apple sauce at a nearby deli. That soothed and comforted me. I dropped out of class when the drama in my life exceeded any drama class that existed in the college catalogue.

My nineteen year old husband was into heavy partying which included leaving me alone every weekend while he smoked pot, drank and pursued other women. I tried to reason with him, but as I would later learn, never fight with an intoxicated person. We physically fought and I gave as good as I got but because he was bigger and stronger, I advertised the black eyes and bruises. I tried to keep him out of the clubs I was too young and scared to enter. When he was home, he preferred hanging out on the corner with his friends and I stopped going out completely.

Though the black eyes were not mentioned, my mother started hating Jose. She was smart and she knew what was happening. She encouraged me to go out when I turned eighteen and slyly said she was more than willing to baby sit. The night life beckoned and I went off like the Pied Piper's children to their doom. I never took drugs or drank. I am very emphatic when innocent. They were not my vices. I didn't sleep with other men, but I danced, flirted and stayed out all night. I even met Jose in one of the clubs where we both were flirting with others. I went up to him and the girl sitting on his lap and made a scene forgetting that I was as guilty as he was. He left with me and we fought on the subway-all the way home.

One day, I went to Central Park with my new friends and we hung out at The Fountain all day. I left and picked up my daughter from my mother's house and she gave me a jar of home made potato salad. When Jose, hung over from his night of partying, demanded his dinner because that was the right of any upstanding Latino husband, I handed him the potato salad in the jar. He ate it with a hateful look on his face. When he was done he threw the jar at me. The jar splintered in pieces and imbedded in my thigh. As the blood poured, I became eerily calm as I always do when faced with real drama. My baby was in the carriage right behind me and though it didn't hit the carriage it could have. It was sobering that he would endanger our baby. When we couldn't stop the profuse bleeding, he called the ambulance against my objections. I thought I deserved to bleed to death so my baby would be given to someone worthier than MM. The police came and grilled us about how the glass entered my leg at an angle. But I stood by my story that it was an accident. They didn't believe me but chose not to arrest Jose. The police were the enemy who would expose the shame that we were the parents from hell. I was used to bad treatment; being abused. It was familiar and I deserved it. At the hospital I was given twelve stitches in one part of my leg and four in the other. Jose knew my calm request for him to leave was dead serious and I helped him pack trying to appease him in some way for having to throw him out.

This time he left without an argument. We separated and I proceeded to go wild over the next few months, and though my agoraphobia was in remission for a while, I would not come away unscathed. The night he left would bring me face to face with death.

I went back with Jose some time after that and we had a son together but the marriage continued to be violent and mad. I didn't love him, I had never loved him and finally, it was more painful to stay than go. He said he loved me and when his drinking and drug taking escalated I knew my plan to escape had been a good one. I worked and saved every penny while he stalked me to three apartments in the Bronx.

My agoraphobia rose and fell in spurts before and after that time, but my children became my main reason for not giving up on life. I took my daughter away from my mother and tried to ignore the fact that my mother's subsequent hospitalization with major depression wasn't my fault.

I was eighteen and I had protected my daughter from both my mother and my husband. My mother was wrong. Maybe I wasn't Mother Theresa but I wasn't Mother MCCREE either.

CHAPTER 18

TROUBLE

There are many signals that your marriage is doomed. Some relationships end with a bang, some with a whimper, but sometimes, one incident brings you over the edge. Your partner seems determined for you to notice some of their outrageous behavior. You see it all with new eyes. Maybe it's something you always accepted with "Hey that's the way he is," or, "Oh, well no one's perfect." But one seemingly normal particular day, they do something, not even the most egregious act they ever pulled, and you say, "That's the final nail in the coffin! I can't take one more moment of this person."

My breaking point with Jose wasn't the drama that brought the police or the police dog to our home. He had been a gentle man when we wed a bit shy, straight from the mountains of Puerto Rico, with a dry sense of humor and he adored me. The problems began when he started smoking pot and drinking more than a skinny man should. I wasn't afraid of him. Well, not until he brought the pit bull home. One morning, I woke up to the sight of "Cujo" dragging a huge chain behind him and barking and growling so loud, the neighbors started coming out of their apartments, not easy in Brooklyn.

Jose smiled and said, "He tried to attack me on my way home, but I made friends with him and now he is ours."

"This is a guard dog," I said. "He belongs to someone."

"Yes, he belongs to the bakery I was 'borrowing' some breakfast from, but now he's ours." Thankfully, Cujo didn't agree and when he saw an open window he jumped out. If I had been able to I would have joined him.

One day, I said, "Joe, I'm worried. Most of the apartments in our building are being robbed at night and I'm alone with Elena and pregnant."

He chuckled, "Don't worry; you're not going to get robbed."

"How do you know?"

After laughing himself silly, he gasped, "Because I'm the robber," taking out a wad of cash to prove his point. "Me, and Chino got a part time job."

My heart started thumping. I was paralyzed with fear. Chino, a half-Chinese, half Puerto Rican boy, I had a mild crush on, was his partner in crime, literally. I started laughing hysterically, he wasn't fazed or realizing, I wasn't right mentally. Nothing fazed him. When he did stumble in with stale beer on his breath and cheap perfume on his body, he ignored my daughter and me.

I hardly noticed he was gone unless there was this kind of drama. I was distracted the whole pregnancy with talk radio, fearfully rereading the book, "Childbirth without Fear" and eating gallons of vanilla ice-cream. He didn't notice or care that I hadn't seen an obstetrician until I was five months along, so terrified of both the internal exam and acknowledging I was pregnant again with a man I never loved but married to get rid of a sick mother. Jose also didn't notice I hardly left the house or when I finally did, started to see a hypnotherapist at Maimonides Hospital in Brooklyn who tried to open me up in all ways, to face my fears.

The day I went into labor, Jose was sleeping off a Thursday night drunk and I stayed awake all night sitting on the living room couch waiting for the three minute contractions that signaled it was time to leave for the hospital. I waited until 11 a.m. Jose was still asleep and though he had to work later that day he was hung-over and passed out. I tried to wake him up but it's even harder to wake up a drunk than win an argument with one.

I told him I was in labor and he finally snarled, "Take the bus to the hospital," so I did.

On the bus, I couldn't suppress a small yelp or gasp when we hit bumps in the road.

"Are you ok?" an older woman wearing a Sari asked. I did notice that the bus riders were more concerned with my well being than my husband. The Indian woman got off the bus with me, escorted my big belly inside the hospital and told an attendant I was in labor.

The next thing I knew, I was hooked up to various machines and intravenous tubes. I was considered high risk because of my overdue date, lack of pre-natal care and profusion of panic attacks.

On my last visit, the doctor warned, "Marilyn, you might need a Cesarean, the baby looks big and I can't examine you properly." I had taken my daughter Elena to my mother's house two weeks earlier. Jose didn't even notice she was gone.

A few hours later, Jose arrived at the hospital resplendent in his bell bottoms, shiny green platform shoes with a hat sitting jauntily on his curly head. He started to bicker with me because our tax refund check had arrived in the mail, and didn't I realize he needed me to sign the check in person because it was in both our names? Didn't I realize he had plans for the weekend and needed money because payday was not until next week? Why was I so selfish to say I was giving birth today when he had a weekend of drinking and fun ahead of him?

The nail wasn't yet in when he found my doctor and demanded my release from the hospital.

The doctor looked at him amazed, "Sir, you wife is giving birth."

"Not NOW", he replied, as the nurse rolled her eyes.

I so wanted to believe that he could release me from the pain I was in and obediently started to remove the tubes that held me tethered to that bed. As I struggled to get up, the nurse gently pushed me back down.

"You aren't going anywhere," she said. "Cash a check," I heard her mumble to herself, "what an idiot."

The doctor walked away as Jose started pleading.

"I'll get her back here in an hour tops," in his once sweet to me Spanish accent.

As my labor progressed to exquisite intensity without the benefit of today's epidural miracle or my husband, I asked for the phone to call my mother. The nurse brought the phone to my bed and dialed. I wanted to tell my mother I was finally in labor.

As I reached for the phone, the nurse hung up. "Your mother said "good luck" she deadpanned.

She went to the sink and wet a towel and brushed my tangled hair away and placed the towel on my forehead saying. "Honey, you got trouble."

I gave birth to my son Jason Luis Rivera at two minutes to noon the next day, March 17, 1972. It had been a difficult birth. I had to go for X-rays twice to make sure he could be delivered vaginally. I was knocked out to give birth and twice I awoke still full of baby. Surely this was a nightmare. When I woke up the third time, he was born, all 7 pounds 8 ounces of beauty. He was Jose in miniature with a full head of curls and long eyelashes. All the nurses fussed over the baby with the head of dark hair and beautiful face. No one came to visit me until the fifth day when I had to leave the hospital.

Jose arrived in the same outfit, smelling like a brewery. "So, you finally had the baby. Now you can cash the check." I was forced to notice the whine in his voice and something else: a distant sound was interrupting the joy of holding my son. It was the sound of that final nail being pounded in the coffin. It went in deep, very deep!

Jan 11

I acted OK, today. I am tired of writing the same old complaints. I had a wonderful dream last night, I saw all my grandchildren and my Marilyn. How I love them. It was so very good that dream that when I woke up Carl at 9 o'clock, I still felt good and told Carl I was going to be OK. How I wish that were true. But going to the clinic and talking, talking about the same old thing my mood didn't last. But I am acting OK. I am going to try to get dressed in the morning and go out. God give me the strength. I met some man that was sick 11 years ago, but he is fine now. He said if he could do it so can I. I hope so. I called the police. They had no news about Angie. It really is Carl's fault for letting him out that day but I wouldn't tell him. How could he know? I should have stopped him. Carl is making me feel worse. He is so worried about Angie that he's acting Ok, is not acting he really is worried. I'm tired of this life and wish I heard some good news. It is 8:15. I have a sore throat. I forced myself to eat a lot of chicken and mashed potatoes. I wish it was with an appetite. I'm tired of forcing myself to eat for Carl's sake. I wish we had some good news. I am an old woman but just 6 months ago I was reading complicated books, the libraries best customer. I have read thousands of books in my lifetime. About 5 book a week. How I loved reading. Please give me back my power of love of reading. Is it wishful thinking? I am waiting for 9 o'clock; Morton Downey on Channel 9. I'm not used to going out anymore. That is why I have the chills and a sore throat. I have this compulsion to write. I hope it goes away with my sickness. I'm tired of doctors and social workers. I want to be as I was before. I never liked to write. I didn't even like to answer letters .I Just loved making shopping lists, taking care of bills, buying with my Visa, balancing my checkbook. I think this writing is good for me the way I am now. But when I feel better I won't. It relaxes me now. What if I didn't know how to write? I used to have a neighbor who didn't and I used to write to her children and fill out forms. She loved me and she was crazy about Elena who I took care of when Marilyn worked. It broke my heart. I had her for the first 7 months when she was born. Then Marilyn took her back when she moved to Bensonhurst. That was 18 years ago. Who ever thought I'd end up like this? I thought the older I got, the wiser I would be. I just asked if it was OK to eat my jello with a sore throat and he got angry. Carl was so happy with Angie knowing he was safe with him. That's all we needed. Goodnight.

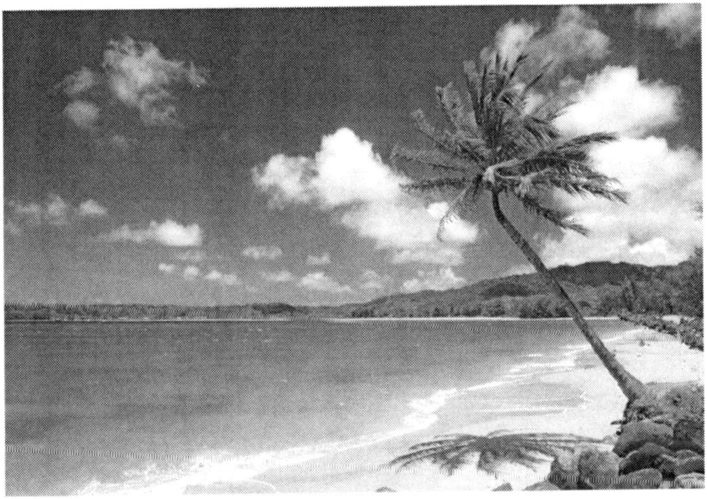

CHAPTER 19

FAR, FAR AWAY

I used to ask my mother what song I should sing and she always said "Far, Far Away." Little did she realize that would become my mantra when I left New York City for good; August 24th on my twenty- fifth birthday.

When I was twelve and watched the movie "South Pacific" for the first time. I made up my mind wherever it was filmed I would find a way to live there. At the end of the movie, the credits read "filmed in Kauai, Hawaii."

"That's my place," I said as my friends laughed. No one was laughing when I packed up my two children, our suitcases and the thousand dollars I had saved in a year and got the hell out of Dodge. My mother sneered and said I would be back in three months. I still live here.

My mother didn't hug me when I left but that was normal because hugging wasn't her way. She didn't show feelings, unless they were critical or angry.

"When I'm sick, I'm nice," she said. Or her favorite: "g-d didn't make us all the same."

If I got a grade of 98 in school, the inevitable "where's the other two points" was asked. When Mrs. Toverasky called me docile on my report card, she exploded with, "Docile! They say that about horses. I'll give her docile!" When I occasionally broke out of my expected substandard behavior, she would be somehow embarrassed.

When I was "Anna" in my 9th grade production of the "King and I", and received a corsage of orchids from the principal and the complement, "Your daughter is going to be famous." She scowled at him and said, "I'll be lucky if she gets to be a secretary." He just stared as I cringed somehow knowing all the accolades I received were fake. I was an imposter. When we walked home, she told me not to get stars in my eyes. I had to realize that I was not pretty enough to be in show business and I would just get hurt. She called it constructive criticism but this raining on my parade was setting me up for deep depression in the future, ironically the same depression she suffered from without the manic phase.

A few years later when I was sixteen, I escaped from her physically into a doomed marriage, but couldn't get away from the anxiety and depression that invaded the deep places inside where boundaries were blurred.

I was twenty four and working as a "utility clerk" in the garment district of New York. This meant I opened up mail and distributed it around the office as well as counting checks in amounts I would never see. Since I was close to Times Square I found a news stand called "Shindler's." On my lunch hour, I poured over papers from around the world. I saved a thousand dollars and with a wing (actually United Airlines Wings) and a prayer, I purchased a one way ticket to Hawaii. The prayer was a pen pal named David Chun, an older man who wrote me letters and offered me a room in his house until I got settled. He told me he wrote angry letters to the editor of the "Honolulu Advertiser" every day, but I wasn't smart enough then to know what a red flag was.

I planned a going away party and told everyone I would live in Waipahu, pronouncing it with the accent on the u instead of the correct ending of pa on Oahu at the time according to the "Honolulu Advertiser" and planned a going away party. My party was a blast. I played Hawaiian music, did a happy dance and played down my mothers doom that Hawaii was full of rats. I was always afraid of mice so I think that was a smart way of getting me to stay home. It didn't work. She called me crazy and I acted the part while playing down the gloom.

But I couldn't fool myself. In the airplane on the way to Hawaii, I had a panic attack. I peered at my face in the bathroom mirror and my mothers tapes played in my ear while my heart pounded and my throat closed. “Pimples, you’re so ugly. No one will ever want you no matter where you go; you will be nothing. You will fail.” I gagged into the sink, hating my bloated red face with the acne scars so visible without my makeup. Wash your face, hotter, hotter, burn those pimples and scars off. The water on the plane was cold but it burned my face nevertheless.

At the Honolulu airport, my game face was on as my pen pal greeted me. He was a shriveled Chinese man with a raspy voice. In his letters I had pictured him as sophisticated and cheerful. He no longer drove so he brought his neighbor, a cute Asian local guy who was very friendly to my children and we went on a mini tour of the Island. I remember the blow hole, a spouting steam of water impossibly coming from a small hole in the ocean. The palm trees at his house seemed to welcome me home. But I had to face a mini ordeal first.

As I know now but didn’t realize then, nothing is for free. He had bought a box of dim sum or what is called “Manapua” in Hawaii. This turned out to be a box of rice cakes and doughy balls with charsiu or roast pig inside. He wanted me to eat. The strange food and my anxiety formed a knot in my stomach and I couldn’t eat enough to satisfy him. He said he had paid five dollars for the box and in 1976 that was a lot of money. My children were so tired I put them in the bedroom to sleep and stayed in the living room to talk to him thinking we could at least have some good conversation which I felt I owed him. He said, “Now we dance” and put on some foxtrot music. His gnarled fingers reached eagerly for me. I told him I was too tired to dance and he became angry. I scurried away to the room before he could protest too much, realizing I had to leave as soon as morning came.

Yet, before I fell asleep, the perfume and magic of the island spoke to me. You made the right choice. You'll heal here. Your children will thrive in this place. The palm trees seemed to nod in agreement. I breathed in my new surroundings and peace descended on me. In that instant, I was safe, happy, and far, far away.

PART 4

THINKING OUTSIDE OF THE BOX

FROM ERROR TO ERROR, ONE DISCOVERS THE ENTIRE TRUTH
SIGMUND FREUD

Jan 12,

It is 12:30 in the afternoon. I am very sick. Oh God, give me peace. What shall I do all day? Carl took the little lady to the doctor. Her face is all swollen. Angie is still missing. I called the police again. They can't do anything. I am waiting for a call from them. I would feel much better if he called for Carl's sake. Carl looks terrible. I have to behave all day. I am not behaving. I wet my hair in cold water again even though I have a sore throat. Please let me die. I can't live anymore. I thought a miracle would happen if I came home from the hospital but it all went wrong.

1. *Angie might be in a critical condition, Carl away all day. Me at home with a cold*
2. *Telephone out of order one week nobody to talk to or get in touch with*
3. *I did not force myself to go out*
4. *I came home sick*

I always fought it. In fact I was out of hospitals for 12 years. Carl is angry with me because I wanted to help Marilyn. He lost his temper and yelled that he couldn't care for me.

The hospital made me worse

Carl came home with lots of food. He seems to think the more I eat the better my head will get. I wish it were true. I HATE food. I'm tired of forcing myself to eat. It's not even 4 o'clock. Help, help, HELP I beg you God. I don't want to write but I know I will.

Here I go again. It's 5:30. I bothered Carl. Not much just a little. Please let me be calm. Give me peace. I am so tired. I wet my hair again 50 times. In cold water and my throat is sore. What's wrong with me, wetting my head? Before I went to the hospital I never did that or wrote or was so sick

I just told Carl I don't believe in God. There is a Jewish song my father used to sing (God knows what he does and he doesn't punish anyone) I don't believe it. I hope nobody reads this lousy diary. I am going to be 74 in May. I hope I get better soon. My hand is tired of writing. I'm going to try to read the paper. In fact, Carl bought 2 papers. He had a good life until Angie and I got sick. He went where he pleased all through our marriage. WHAT A POOR EXCUSE FOR A WOMAN I WAS! I should have gone to work. I never liked to work but I did for about 15 years.

It is 6:30. Ok let me die now. Don't let me suffer anymore. Carl gave me an alcohol rub. I say I don't believe in God but I keep on praying. I can't fight. I have to go to the hospital which I fear. Tonight I can't stop writing. I am trying to be calm. I don't want to write anymore. I have writer's cramp. I will say goodnight. I am so tired.

CHAPTER 20

TAKING A BREAK

It is a brilliant Hawaiian day and I am lying on a deserted sidewalk in Honolulu. I don't want to live. I drag my feet like a heavy anchor that seems to invade my being and drops me to the ground.

I think it's about my second husband Junior not coming home for a week, but the pain is so intense and the depression so exhausting I pray for death. There seems to be glue stuck to the bottom of my flip flops, but I finally get up and struggle to a phone to call my friend Doni.

"I want to kill myself."

"Go home, you'll feel better."

"I'm in the street, help me."

"You'll be alright, just go home."

"I can't."

"You can get up, just try. Go eat something, you're probably dehydrated."

I went home and ate melted vanilla ice cream until I passed out in a sugar coma. Sugar can medicate as well as Prozac. I didn't want to die, I just wanted relief.

Castle hospital is a Seventh Day Adventist hospital nestled between the Koolau Mountains on the windward wet green side of the island of Oahu. It prides itself as being a holistic healing place treating the patient's physical, mental and spiritual needs. By the time I was thirty five, it had been my home away from home three times. I prided myself that I always was admitted on a voluntary basis; not taken by force after a suicide or murder attempt although I came close on my first stay.

I was never privy to the locked section with the padded cells and big burly Samoan orderlies who made sure you didn't kill yourself with the strings of your open hospital gown. But I saw all these people after their initial crisis was over. We had lunch and group therapy and walked together on our outings to the beach.

It was like kindergarten again, only better, complete with arts and crafts, dancing and primal screams. We were given medications that weren't effective with breakfast and our doctors visited us in our rooms once a day. In between, kindness and sternness were handed out in equal doses. The vegetarian food was to clean out the garbage in our intestines. The garbage inside was harder to cure.

I met many women like me who had been betrayed by a significant other. There was Deana, a thirty something nurse who had dated a married guy for five years and believed that he would leave his wife until she was confronted by the eight month pregnant woman in a supermarket.

"How can that happen, she asked me, when they never had sex?"

She took an overdose of pills and called the scoundrel to say goodbye. When she woke up she was in the above padded cell. I also met Sharon, a military wife who had been married for five years who had just arrived in Hawaii where her husband told her, he didn't love her anymore. She tried to hang herself in the closet.

The woman I felt closest to was Olga, a Swedish woman married to an older rich man, who adored her. She had such a beautiful soul, we became fast friends. He had gone on a business trip and left her alone with his naughty teen son and she went on a drinking binge and ended up getting in her car in her nightgown and crashing into the garage door. When the police came, she tried to stab herself.

My first trip to Castle Hospital coincided with the birth of my son and my second husband Junior's infidelity. He cleaned, ironed and cooked, and I felt taken care of. So

I promptly fell in love and never saw the immature player he really was. I created him in my mind. We had just bought a house, and he convinced me to try to get pregnant; that he would help me throughout the process. He helped me by having an affair with a married waitress at the restaurant. He was the cook, how tacky. Thankfully, I was innocent of this until the birth of my son. I had my suspicions but believed him; that he was working double shifts, helping his brother build a house and too tired to drive to the country where we lived. I even didn't catch on when two Filipino waitresses visited me in my ninth month telling me a story of two married employees who were having an affair at the restaurant. They gave me significant looks that I didn't catch. My best friend Ana doesn't call me "Sherlock" for naught. They told me this "disgraceful man had even taken this woman to visit his family. I felt sorry for the poor woman and never realized it was me. My anxiety about giving birth was so great I didn't catch the significance until my son was six months old and my husband brought home a new red Camaro that he said his friend allowed him to drive. He became blatant in his infidelity and didn't touch me for six months. His girlfriend would pick him up at the house in the morning and there would be whispered conversations on the phone at night. He even let me speak to her saying she was a co-worker he was "helping" with the new menu and job. The job was the horizontal kind and I became obsessed with his affair.

To say I felt betrayed is too mild. To say I became hysterical cannot convey my rage and anger at him. To say I was dangerous to myself and my children would be more accurate. I became an insane detective and followed him on the bus, babe in arms. I do not drive so I hid in bushes behind the restaurant to catch him with her. When his sister told me she was a waitress in the restaurant, I went there and she actually seated me. She was the hostess and I didn't even guess. I was told she was Hawaiian but I was determined to find out who my rival was. She was a goddess and I was an ugly sad bitch. In reality she was older, white and plain. Our fantasies often betray us.

One morning, early in the affair, he called me early in the morning and said he loved me after being out all night. I knew something was up but I was still in denial. This was the first time he had slept with her. His sex habits, the few times we did it, changed too. He wanted me on top and to say, "He Haw, the rodeo is good." (Men, don't do this if you cheat) It's a give away every time even if your wife is as clueless and distracted as I was.

This farce came to a head when on his day off he went off to work after receiving an obvious call from "her." I knew it wasn't true and when he left I ran a mile to call his job because our phone wasn't working, leaving my baby alone in the house. His boss Lei, told me that Eve, the co-worker was also absent that day. Wait, where was my baby? I panicked and called a friend to come to my house to help, knowing I was officially insane. I wandered in a fog throughout Honolulu thinking simultaneously of murder and suicide. When I arrived home, Junior was there and admitted he had been fooling around for a long time with Eve. I threw all his clothes in the street. His parting words to my eleven year old son were, "You're a man now, take care of your mother." I wanted to kill him for that.

I was admitted in the hospital three days later. He refused to take care of our children; he was too involved with cheating and drinking. The authorities wouldn't let my friend Stephanie take care of them, so they were put in foster care for three weeks and abused. My eldest daughter was given the task of taking care of the baby while the "foster mother" sat on her fat ass inside. They were forced outside in the noon Hawaiian heat, and one day my daughter went a long walk seeking shade and the foster mother got nervous and looked for her and screamed in her face. At night roaches walked over them as they slept on a futon on the floor. My husband, this person who was my rock, disintegrated into dust and the esteem that I had invested in him and not myself fell like a dead weight on a feather.

When I entered the hospital, I was given a physical exam and the doctor asked me about the bruises all over my body.

"Who beat you", he said.

"No one," I said truthfully as he looked at me with disbelief.

Then I remembered,

"Oh," I said and kept quiet.

I had kept questioning my husband about the evidence I found, like credit card receipts with Vodka gimlets and beers and the perfume he reeked of. When he couldn't answer he would throw me to the floor and kick me until I was quiet and still. But I couldn't stop the questions and he couldn't stop beating me.

I was told I needed to rest, get a restraining order (they weren't fooled) and not worry about anything; but resting in a psychiatric ward is not easy. My roommate was an anorexic nun who had a habit of staying up all night saying rosaries. I have an aversion to sleeping with strangers so I started hanging out with the cool night staff that included a cute Black guy I promptly fell in lust with. We talked about life, how it can make you crazy and he sang to me until I got sleepy.

Being in a loony bin takes away some of the pressures of life but not all and I was ridiculed and bullied there too. I found that life inside can be a microcosm of life anywhere.

"Love looks not with the eyes but with the mind." Our group therapy session had begun and our therapist looks at me with meaning." He believes Shakespeare holds the answers to our broken souls. .The girl who throws cereal in my hair every day speaks.

"Her left eye always looks at the door."

She started laughing at her joke. Our leader says nothing but looks sorry. So am I.

A guy who had just come from the locked ward was walking in the back of me and stage whispers that I look like Linda Blair, when her head was spinning around in the Exorcist. He laughs and I remember my mothers tape. "Pimple faced bastard." That's why my husband left. I wasn't pretty enough to keep him. I am ugly. I am worthless.

One evening, a young Samoan man was admitted and wandered in my room. His girlfriend had dumped him and he had attempted suicide. He had just been let out of the locked section and I felt his loss. He started kissing me and we fell to the bed until a nurse came in and separated us. We were both lost and his desperation was so familiar. I wanted to save him and myself and at the time, sex was the only remedy. The next day he didn't remember me.

In group therapy that day, I opened up about how lonely I felt in my lonely house with my new baby rocking him all alone while my husband fucked his girlfriend. I cried as I told them I listened to Phil Collins "One more night" and how I wanted to die if my husband didn't want me anymore. As an exercise in trust, we were instructed to fall backwards in the arms of someone we think we trust. I fell backwards into the Samoan boy's arms and from that day I started to heal...

I went home soon after that, got a divorce and married Manny who said he adored me and would help me raise my four children. He was funny and he made me laugh until his addictions made me cry.

I went back to the Castle two more times with panic disorder, hysteria, and depression, fell out of love with Junior, who ended up marrying another woman, not Eve. It would take me many years before I realized no man is worth dying for. I thought then after breaking down, the only direction was up, but I would be sadly mistaken.

CHAPTER 21

AGORAPHOBIA, ANXIETY, HYPOCHONDRIA OH MY!

I am twenty-three years old and in the emergency room trying to convince the ER doctor, I have a brain tumor. I had been crying in my closet for weeks, with a persistent headache and a bump on my head that I discovered while trying to rub the pain away. Why doesn't the headache go away? One morning I wake up with a terror that is so strong it forces me to face the truth that I am dying and sends me to the one place I try to avoid at all costs; a hospital.

The doctor looks at me after giving me a rudimentary brain test. "Walk a straight line, close your eyes and touch your finger to your nose and straight out," he said while peering in my eyes with a light.

"Look at me, he says, you don't have a brain tumor and you are not dying, Brain tumors usually happen when you are under twelve or over forty. That bump on your head is the fontanel, the baby's soft spot that hardens into a bump. What you do have is a severe case of acne, and hypochondria, you need to see a dermatologist and a therapist."

Great, my diagnosis is acne which I knew I had, and hypochondria which I don't understand.

I have been to emergency rooms many, many times since that day. I have frightened many doctors by crying hysterically when I am asked then bullied to take a blood test or a mammogram. I just know it will reveal some horrible disease I have- like hypochondria.

Later, when I lived in Kauai during my daughter's senior year, the room spun so fast I thought I was some crazy amusement park ride. I could only sleep on one side and thought I was dying. My doctor at the time told me it would go away and it did. What they failed to address was the tooth infection that caused the dizziness and they anxiety they called hypochondria. I have been in such scary places in my mind that even my closet couldn't contain the fear.

I am in the health center complaining yet again about a pain in my shoulder that won't go away. Dr. McCain explains it is a torn ligament but I am sure I am dying. I would continue to have stiff muscles and pain all over my body that were eventually diagnosed as fibromyalgia but that day when Dr. McCain suggested a blood gas test that would confirm I wasn't seriously ill, I became hysterical and screamed and cried so violently, I could see the fear and shock in his eyes. I left without the dreaded test but Dr. McCain told me he was worried that one day I could potentially have a serious problem with my health and not be diagnosed.

I also shocked a whole board of psychiatry. I was asked by the local mental health center if I would speak at their monthly meeting, I had no idea what they had in mind. They started to ask me questions about my being hand fed until age twelve and some of the names I had been called on a daily basis. My answers were told in a monotone voice because I truly had not connected my anxiety attacks to my past. But when I saw their faces in pity and disbelief, I felt shame. I had been set up. I knew they pitied me, but I really didn't know why. I felt like I was being abused in some way but I didn't understand it. This feeling of betrayal and abuse was a familiar one, but until that time, never with a health professional. As I left the office, I heard them start talking all at once and I knew something I had said was wrong and I was stupid and guilty. Had I betrayed my mother as my psychologist had just betrayed me?

I recently told my eighty five year old aunt that when I had pneumonia that my mother hung the phone up on me. Her first reaction was to laugh. She thought I was kidding or telling some kind of weird joke. She couldn't or didn't want to believe that my mother could do that. She again repeated how much my mother had loved me; how she told her I was her life.

"Auntie, I know she loved me, but she hurt me too."

It was time to tell my truth. I was twenty eight, very sick, hospitalized with severe pneumonia.

I was scared and called my mother and said. "Mom I'm scared, I'm in the hospital with pneumonia," and that's when she hung up on me.

I called back thinking we had lost the connection and in her meanest voice she snarled, "Don't ever call me up with bad news."

My mother must have guessed but never discussed all my bad news. After her death, my letters to her came back to me and the sunny lying letters hiding the ambulance runs, the anxiety, and finally my agoraphobia were hiding in; how happy the family was and sounds strangely childlike.

"Mommy I would say, you will never guess what happened today, the family went on a picnic and the baby walked for the first time." I didn't tell her I wasn't there for that event because I was so dizzy I couldn't even walk.

My hypochondria were symptoms of anxiety and there came a point I hardly went to doctors at all. I would suffer in my closet.

Later I found out patients with hypochondria rarely avoid doctors. They want all the tests to prove they are right. I was too scared for the tests that would prove I had more than hypochondria. I was so scared of death.

Later on, I had a bad result on a mammogram and had to have a biopsy which turned out to be ok. But I ended up in an emergency room before the day of the biopsy with a panic attack.

A wise doctor examined me and looked me in the eyes and said, "I am almost positive that you don't have cancer."

I didn't, but I had the second mammogram and when that came out benign, never went back, afraid to go through the severe mental torture again.

I finally got the point. I learned my symptoms were classic signs of an anxiety disorder. This disorder masked the real issues I had to deal with to get well. I was in trouble and it was easier to focus on the panic attacks than the traumas I had experienced in my life.

The fear of a brain tumor was a way of diverting my attention from the really scary thoughts and memories that were protected by fear. But until I faced the real monster, a bump on my head, a false positive mammogram or a blood test would keep my brain dizzy and the reality wouldn't bubble to the surface. I wasn't yet ready to deal with that dilemma so my mental illness would have to get much worse before I was ready to face the fear which was scarier than death.

CHAPTER 22

GROUP THERAPY

You know you have a problem with food when you have a tug of war with your ten year old son, over a plum. I was a single parent and money was tight and we were living on hot dogs and macaroni and cheese but a food bank had given us five plums. My son had eaten his and grabbed mine and attempted to run away. I ran after him like my life depended on it and at almost two hundred pounds running was no easy task. I caught him and we had a tug of war. Back and forth, the plum passed between us while my other three kids cheered us on. That juicy plum would be mine and my mouth watered in anticipation. He had youth and energy on his side; I had food addiction and desperation on mine... I won. When I took that first bite of the plum in front of him, triumphant in my win, he started crying.

"You big butt punk" but I couldn't stop eating it. The next day I went to Overeaters Anonymous.

I have never been a group person. It's not that I don't like groups; it's that groups don't like me. It's not even that I couldn't pretend to be interested in the most disjointed confessions; I listened intently as everyone told their stories. We weren't allowed to mention a particular food or give or get advice and this seemed to defeat the purpose for me. I wanted advice. I needed to be shamed to stop my bizarre behavior. I listened to all the stories about higher powers and abstinence not really understanding. But my plum shame was as huge as I was and I had to speak. As I told my story, calling the plum, a piece of fruit, I started to notice a strange reaction. The serious man, who had told with pride his long story of recovery and abstinence, was smiling. As his moustache quivered, I looked around and other members were trying hard to hold back their laughter.

Finally one lady gasped and hid her head but not before I saw her mouth wide with silent contractions of hysteria. Great! I was a hit with this somber group. I took their materials and went back to the meeting the next week but noticed if I started to speak, some one else would chime in until the meeting ended. I was never again allowed to give them a reason to shame themselves. When they spoke to me, only if pressed, I realized that yet again I was ostracized by a group. I had to find another way to deal with this madness.

I should have listened to my ex- boyfriend Hiroki, who said there was something about me that makes men eager to push me over a cliff. I didn't believe him because he had severe anger explosive disorder meaning he blew up like a volcano if you breathed the wrong way. But in this instance, he makes a good point. In every group situation, something goes terribly wrong.

I joined a woman's liberation/therapy group in the late 70's. I was young and was seeking help with my depression and anxiety. I was quiet for weeks listening and waiting for the right time to speak.

The minute I opened my mouth and said, "I feel sad and I don't know why, you know," an older woman started to harass me.

She turned to me irate and slurred, "Don't you know it's a sign of low self- esteem when you say "you know" after every sentence.

What insight!

I turned to the moderator for help but her inexperience and youth had her nervously changing the subject.

After the meeting, she took me aside and said, "Ignore her, she's an alcoholic and jealous of young women." I went back one more time, where I saw her eyes watching me and waiting for me to speak, I started thinking she might be a witch, and I mean a real one. When I didn't meet her "crazy eyes" she ranted.

"Women with low self esteem really bug me, and I want to shake them silly."

I quit the group that night, you know. Oops!

I still tried joining groups. I tried Weight Watchers, but gained weight because of my boredom about talking about how you can eat a can of spinach while driving if you get desperate. I hate spinach and don't drive.

Two single's groups rejected me for being too young and then too old. A mental health self- esteem workshop went horribly wrong. An aspiring comedian behaved fine in the morning while discussing his goals and dreams. But In the afternoon his comedy turned into tragedy, when he locked us all in the room and starting ranting and raving, his mental illness not letting him handle a full day of self- esteem. I had a full blown panic attack right then and there. I hate being closed in unless it's self- imposed. The ambulance had to take us both away to the emergency room where we laid in separate gurneys in the hospital hallway looking at each other. Comedy indeed!

Even in an inpatient group therapy session, a nun turned on me for leaving my kids to have a nervous breakdown. She was there against her will by the Catholic Church for thinking an angel was in love with her and refusing to eat. In that group, an Anglican minister said to me "You have smart eyes."

As I momentarily basked in the praise, a teenager crack addict said "Yea, I noticed her eyes are crossed."

The nun piped up, "she must have the devil inside".

I try to analyze what I do wrong. Maybe it's my personality that gets on groups nerves. I talk a bit too fast; I'm a tad too eager to answer the unanswerable and a bit too happy to be anywhere. But somehow groups always leave a bitter taste in my mouth, like that plum.

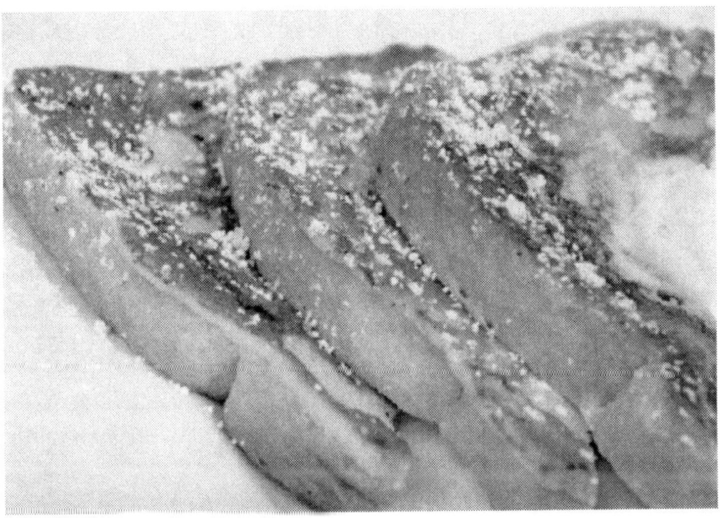

CHAPTER 23

WHAT I DID FOR LOVE (OF FRENCH TOAST)

My mother made the best French toast in the whole wide world. I watched her on the weekends while she dipped the white bread in the mixture of eggs and milk. Her recipe wasn't fancy. She never added vanilla or cream or maple syrup and butter. That was for goyin (non Jews) but I would learn about those lovely additions later when I was free. But the milk was always whole and the eggs just tasted better in the fifties. If I was there watching, she always explained her recipe; she knew a good audience when she saw one.

"Always get the oil hot in the big iron pan before putting the bread in. Then fry them to brown perfection. Don't undercook them and set out the cinnamon and sugar before mixing them together. I would discover maple syrup later. Weekends were when I was allowed to eat French toast and not the horrid cereal and soft boiled egg she hand-fed me. In the summer, I could ask for it every day, so I was especially excited. So enthusiastic and often did I speak of my mothers' French toast that sometimes my friends showed up for breakfast. To my mother's credit, she always fed them. She was as proud as I was.

I was never allowed to cook, or even do dishes though I always offered, and my father being old-school Latino, expected girls to learn housekeeping and cooking. "Teach her something," he would yell in his booming voice.

My mother would yell back, "Her job is studying; she's going to marry a rich man, not like me." I would ignore them as I dipped the French toast in the sweet mixture and the custardy inside hit my palate. I couldn't hear the fighting; I was in French toast heaven.

The portions in our house were huge, and I was expected to eat all my food because some kid I didn't know in some country was starving. We ate huge steaks so rare, blood dripped from them. My father told me the blood would make me strong. With the steak were plates of rice and beans, platters of potatoes, and mountains of tostones. Meat was the cornerstone of our diet. My mother had been through the great depression and my father had almost starved to death in Puerto Rico, so food was very important in our family. We rarely ate vegetables and when my mother thought I had to have spinach, she cooked it to death and mixed it with mashed potatoes with butter and milk because she guessed right that I would hate it. We sometimes had a limp salad with iceberg lettuce drowned in bad oil. Liver was served once a week and was cooked to death, but I gagged it down because leaving food was a sin. My mother did most of the cooking in my early years. But, when my father was home Monday through Wednesday, he cooked (cocina criolla) Puerto Rican specialties, like battered and fried dried cod and pork chops marinated in vinegar and garlic and fried in its juicy sauce (yum).

Everything was served with rice and beans because my father said; no matter what you ate it wasn't a meal to him or any other Puerto Rican without rice and beans. My father's favorite part was called the "Pegau" which means sticky in English. In Puerto Rico they put oil in the bottom of the rice pot and it fries and sticks the end of the rice to the pot. This bottom held the part he craved and though it was thought of as poverty food and it is considered an insult to serve it to a guest in Puerto Rico, he held it above all food. I still remember him crunching the Pegau and the look of joy on his face. I tasted it and though it was crunchy it was too oily for me. He also loved canned pears, and the nights he was at our house for dinner he would open the huge can of pears and ate it with his blue eyes shining like a five year old. He said in Puerto Rico when he was growing up the government would distribute canned pears only at Christmas. He associated canned pears with being rich.

My father was like a rock star, he was illusive and everyone tried to get a piece of him. He loved life and had survived a big hurricane in the 1930's, clinging to a tree and was so poor as a kid, that he had to go to school barefoot and almost died when he stepped on a nail. His one pair of shoes was for church only. He would offer me some of his bowl of pears and I always accepted. I felt honored to share his joy and pears. It was a long time before I realized I was not crazy about canned pears but food has always been more to me than just nourishment. It has power to resurrect the past and nourish and medicate my soul.

I knew I was different in my desire for food very young. Our seventh grade class had lunch at 11:10 a.m. The free lunch was truly disgusting but at 11 a.m. the hunger pangs would start and I would start watching the clock with anxiety hoping it would be something recognizable, but whatever it was I ate it. Most of the time it smelled like old socks, and grease, but I was too hungry to turn it down. The few lucky students who brought sandwiches were looked on with envy by the rest of us. Imagine! Chips and soda both of which my mother never bought, because we couldn't afford anything in addition to the huge meat filled menus we ate. I was always so hungry and never gained weight even with the amount of food I was eating. When my cousin and I went out to a deli in Flatbush Brooklyn, where she had moved to, they would order a large French fries and I would eat most of them

"How do you stay slim eating so much?" her friends would ask me, like going to delis was a frequent occasion for me. Not! I was so hungry I couldn't stop eating the French fries and being slim made it almost acceptable, except for the ketchup dripping down my chin.

Although I wasn't gossiped about in Flatbush for my weight, boys told my cousin if I had nice clothes and good skin, they would ask me out because I had a nice shape. I never minded because hanging out with Cindy who treated me like a sister was worth anything. She was a star and I was Cousin Marilyn and accepted by her friends because of that.

Later, I would discover favorite foods like potato pancakes dipped in apple sauce, macaroni and cheese, and would always bring two huge pastrami sandwiches to work. I was thirteen, almost fourteen, when I had my first part-time job and earned my first paycheck of thirty dollars. I made $1.25 cents an hour. I gave my mother most of the money but kept a few dollars for my treats which was potato chips and an orange drink. I was always hungry. I was teased because I ate grown men under the table and stayed thin, for awhile that is. I never had the chance to eat as much as I wanted, which was all the food in the world. I didn't eat cookies, chips and soda because it wasn't in the house, but the binges had started when I had money and access to food. What was I hungry for?

I have expended much energy in my devotion of French toast. Around the time of the plum incident, I had a favorite French toast restaurant in Woolworth at Nicolette Mall, downtown Minneapolis. Minneapolis in not the best place to eat French toast, they specialize in pancakes, which also became one of my binge foods, but I had made it my job to find a decent French toast in Minnesota and this was it, comparable to my favorites in New York. It is amazing how you can spoil this simple but succulent dish by not soaking the bread enough or using the freshest ingredients. Woolworth made the most succulent breakfasts which included an egg skillet my daughter ordered and of course french toast for me. The only problem was they ended breakfast at the unseemly hour of 11 a.m. At 11:01 a.m. almost like Cinderella's night of excitement, you were out of luck.

When I took my daughter to her orthodontist on weekdays, I would always ask for a morning appointment, but inevitably would have to wait and I nervously watched the door for her exit. At 10:45 a.m., I would literally run out of the office, to the shock of the Minnesota school of dentistry, not waiting to make another appointment. I would then say "run" and we would run as fast as we could the few blocks to the restaurant, which wasn't easy on my 193 pound body. Somehow we got there 10.59 and I was always ready in my mind with the excuse we were seated by 11:00, if asked. We never were. I would then order out of breath as my daughter now reminds me "two, two, two orders of French toast," my daughter would add, "and a skillet." She was afraid I would forget her order. Even at twelve, she knew the extent of my French toast obsession.

New York is one of the French toast capitals of the United States and Minnesota is the breakfast capital. The lumberjack pancake breakfasts started with the farmers and pioneers who needed the calories to withstand the hard work and the harsh winters. So I searched in Minnesota for the perfect French toast. They made excellent pancakes but their French toast was mostly inedible. They didn't soak the bread long enough and cooked it either too long or not long enough leaving you with a dry hard piece of bread or a raw egg, that even the best maple syrup couldn't disguise. Then I found "The place." It was Woolworths in downtown Minneapolis and no matter how poor I was I compulsively ate there at least twice a week.

One day, I had a particularly embarrassing encounter with a no no-nonsense waitress who had probably worked there for eternity. She had a hairnet and a face that could only be described as hatchet like. She knew that I somehow didn't belong there; my blonde hair didn't fool her. I was "different" as Minnesotans say in "Minnesota nice" which is sometimes not nice at all.

"I don't take shorthand" she snapped, then walked away, as my daughter hid her head in shame. She shares my love for food, however and wasn't too ashamed to order her "skillet."The breakfast skillet was a monster meal cooked with eggs and bacon and served in the iron pan it was cooked in.

When my French toast came and was thrown unceremoniously at me, I smiled at her and said "thank you" with dignity and as slow as I could. It was my fast talking and high anxiety that had tipped her off. But hatchet face kept glaring at us and it caused my daughter to start laughing uncontrollably and it was contagious. My French toast obsession remains part of my life. Last year, a trip to New York refueled my ardor. I charted known and recommended breakfast places like a general mapping out a war. My eldest daughter, Elena, accompanied me every day to a different place where every day, I ordered French toast and rated it in a book. The only difference is, now I only ask for one order and eat it slowly, savoring every bite.

Elena would say, "Again, the French toast?" I tasted a bit of whatever she ordered but nothing does it for me like the moist wonder that is French toast perfection. I enjoy it just as much as I always have and just eat it in smaller portions as I do now with most food.

In Mary Anne Cohen's excellent healing book, "French Toast for Breakfast" which is not a cookbook but a book perfectly illuminating how to "make peace with emotional eating." She writes, "I have been struck by the number of my patients who have expressed to me a yearning for French toast for breakfast. They seldom satisfied this yearning because it seemed like such a forbidden treat."

It isn't just a treat to me. It's my mother's love. That's what I was hungry for.

CHAPTER 24

MAN, YOU DON'T GIVE YOUR COAT AWAY IN MINNESOTA

Two men speaking outside the "Sharing and Caring Shelter" in Minneapolis

Every place has a distinctive smell. Hawaii's fragrance is sweet tropical blossoms, salt air and coconut tanning oil. Minnesota's is furniture polish, freshly manicured lawns, and popcorn.

I came to Minnesota in the middle of summer wearing sandals and a sundress which shows either a weird optimism or plain stupidly. It was cold. The hotel room was immaculate. The Scandinavian and German's love of cleanliness and diligence seemed to say, "Yuh shure, you bettcha," you betta listen to the rules.

I was good at following rules, but the college I went to Minnesota for didn't have any or I should say not the conventional ones. They took all my community college credits that I had amassed during my ten years of taking one course every semester in Hawaii.

Metropolitan State University of Saint Paul Minnesota had a good reputation and best of all excellent financial aid. I had four kids but I seized the opportunity and once again I was on the road, ill prepared for what would be the worst Minnesota winter in fifty years.

Met State encourages students to design their own degrees and faculty and student's team up to accomplish this. The best part for me was not being forced to go to class most of the time. I could stay home in my Honeywell heated apartment and work at my own speed. This suited my agoraphobia just fine. It's also a way to learn how to be self- directed and focused.

What I didn't plan on was the stunning winter and how to support four children on financial aid and a part time job. Details, always the devil in the details.

I didn't own a coat. I had stopped in New York City from Hawaii to see my parents and my mother exploded, "Carl, she's crazy."

I agreed and shouted "North by Northwest," always playing the fool to both appease her and do what I pleased. This was my chance at what my family told me was impossible, to get my college degree. My professors at the community college in Hawaii had told me I was smart and for the first time in my life, I believed it.

I had done my homework and found out that Bloomington, a southern suburb of Minneapolis had the best schools so we rented a cheap apartment which I later learned was the location of a murder. But to me it just looked like every other building in the neighborhood; Red brick and carpeted hallways smelling of rug cleaner and blueberry muffins.

We snuggled in the three room apartment and my kids started school. I took my son Jonas to third grade at a red brick schoolhouse and a kind teacher greeted us at the front door and welcomed him by name.

"This is like, Leave it to Beaver," my son remarked, and it was.

My daughter was not as lucky on her first day of school. She was the only student with tan skin in this very white suburb and was greeted with "How," a reference to her possibly being Native American. She said, "How what?" Unknowingly we had picked a very conservative suburb. Minnesota's reputation as a liberal and to some a socialist state hid a sinister side. Native and Black Americans were especially looked down upon by some. Since I am white, I heard the "N" word for the first time in my life used in a bad way, and other words for American Indians that didn't make sense to me. I didn't belong in Bloomington. I wore a hat instead of just earmuffs on cold days and talked too fast for the slow talkers there. If you didn't belong in Bloomington they said "She's different," not a compliment I would learn.

I went to a supermarket on my first day there and asked where the soda isle was. The old man working there started at me for a full thirty seconds before slowly saying, "Are you from back East?" I said, "No, West," and when I went to the isle he had pointed to saw the tons of baking soda. I was taught soda was "Pop" and if I wanted a coke, I had to say that, "you bet" another Minnesota saying.

Minneapolis has the largest Native American population of any American city. "Minisota" means "sky tinted water" in the Native Indian Dakota language. Although we both found friends and a decent life, both of us would gain weight and become even more obsessed with food here. Candy stores were everywhere and milk was dispensed in machines like soda machines in fast food restaurants. "Would you like pie with that?" smiling waitresses asked at the end of every meal and all you can eat buffets were a favorite hangout for the obese.

In a few years I found out it was true that no one should eat all you can eat. Five years in Minnesota would not only leave me with permanent arthritis but a sweet tooth that would rival Charlie and his whole chocolate factory.

When winter came, I found out coats were expensive and since I am short and stout in a Latina big butt way, not a Minnesota apple shaped way, I could not find a coat that fit me that was also affordable.

I went to the local church and they were stunned to learn I had come to Minnesota without a coat. I thought the coat they gave me was divine; with down feathers and a hood with fake fur that hid my face. What could be better than that?

My first day wearing it, and an old couple stared at me and I distinctly heard the old man say. "Ma, was that a girl or a boy?" As usual I couldn't figure out if the comment was a compliment or insult because I was almost forty. I didn't care because I was warm which believe me in Minnesota is your main goal.

I soon got in trouble financially and was forced to look for an even cheaper apartment. I found out, taking care of four children on financial aid proved close to be impossible but that Minnesota's Lutheran roots had a safety net for those in poverty.

I heard of a place called "Sharing and Caring" that might help with a rental deposit on a cheaper place.

I had an appointment with a social worker at the homeless shelter and was told to be there at nine in the morning. The nature of my particular agoraphobia makes this very difficult. I could go across the country with less anxiety than having to be on time across town. I was as nervous as a cat about to be tossed in a bathtub when I left the house with my eleven year old daughter Junette. We took the bus from Bloomington to downtown Minneapolis, passed Prince's former club, "First Avenue" and crossed the bridge to where Sharing and Caring is located just as it started to pour. I can't make it through the purple rain; I thought as we trudged across deserted streets, my stomach knotted with anxiety and hunger.

We entered the huge room filled with whole families eating at tables. There was also a long line of mostly men waiting for the hot donuts and coffee.

A loudspeaker droned on "Mothers' keep your children with you. Mothers keep your children with you." The voice had no inflection, just a monotonous drone that communicated hopelessness and poverty. My daughter knew we were going to Woolworth's restaurant later for breakfast; I always had money for my French toast fix. At first she was scared by the scene but soon couldn't resist the smell of hot pastry and entered the donut line. I joined her because as a mother I had to keep my children with me.

Just then in a corner of the room, I saw a sight I will never forget. A cheerful yet serene woman kneeled down in front of men of all races; some with sores festering on their filthy feet. She was washing their feet like she was Mary, the sister of Martha and Lazarus and they were Jesus. She then gave them clean socks to put on, her face shone with a word more intimate than kindness.

I didn't know if I was still on planet earth but this was no ordinary place. The look of love she had for those men who were the forgotten, the unwanted, and the angry; was evident in the care she took with her task. I felt as if I had left planet earth as I had previously known it and maybe was in the presence of an angel.

Her name is Mary Jo Copeland and she started the Sharing and Caring charity in 1981. She is known as the street mother or "urban saint." She has been featured in magazines and on Dateline. But that day I only knew her as someone who saw something beautiful in everyone and had a lesson to teach me about compassion and unconditional love. I didn't know then she was Roman Catholic, a mother of twelve children and was raised with abuse distain and in poverty. I only knew I was in the presence of unconditional love; something I had never experienced...

I left after my appointment with a deposit check in my hand and a strange feeling. I was only told to give love to others and expect nothing in return.

I would have liked to end this story saying I changed that day and never felt the need to be a prisoner in my house, or have a panic attack; but that wouldn't be true. Mental illness is not that simple.

I will say I remember the words of the men talking outside. One had no coat to protect him against the bitter day and he was saying he had given his coat to his cousin who had just arrived from Chicago.

The other man said to him, "Hey man, you crazy. You don't give your coat away in Minnesota." I belonged here, I thought. I was no better or worse than anyone there. I felt dignity in the face of poverty and mental illness. It was in the face of the woman/Angel who washed homeless men's feet and fed hungry people. That morning at our breakfast spot, I left some French toast over on my plate. For once I was satiated and at peace with my swollen body. We left the restaurant and as I pulled my coat tight around me and held my daughters hand, I knew I had learned something that day about dignity and self-respect. I was judging a place: Minnesota by a few people instead of the generosity of the Minnesotans who helped me in my first step to a new life. But the most important lesson I learned that day was to never give my coat away in Minnesota.

CHAPTER 25

THINKING OUTSIDE THE BOX

"Where's mom?" Jonas asks.

"In her boxes," my daughter Elena says. She is cool and matter of fact to her six year old brother, because she has experienced my many years spent hiding in closets with my boxes. I've always been lucky to have had large closets in all my homes. My favorite closet was in Minnesota where I lived while going to college. It was a walk in closet with a dressing room attached to my bedroom. It was literally a cocoon within a cocoon. I ate my meals there, read books and even slept always leaning my head against a box.

There was no collecting or organizing going on in that closet. My head was as jumbled as the few boxes in there. Although containing photos, letters, and journals, I was unable to do more than take them all out and put them back in the same place. I've had reveries in that closet and cried until the boxes were so soaked with tears I almost threw them out. Yet, I felt safe in my boxes in the closet. I was a child again, before the yelling began and no one bothered me there or expected me to do anything. I was free of noise, drama and responsibility. I missed weeks of the blaring television, kids fighting for the last slice of pizza, and the loud swearing rap that my son listened to. But I also missed out on the good stuff, the normal life of a single parent. To my credit, I always came out of the closet when asked. My children and I bonded over the fantasies that ruled my life. We planned many trips we wouldn't take until many years later. We read and reread books on Disneyland until we all felt we had been there. We planned all the rides they wanted to go on, places they wanted to eat and even complicated daily itineraries.

I would always sleep with my children and we all remember the clinking of my ice in the water glass as they clung to my nightgown while we climbed the stairs to my bedroom.

When I was a new mother, still a teenager, my daughter would ask me, "Do you love me mommy?"

"Yes, will you ever leave me?"

"Never, mommy, I'll never leave you," she answered seriously.

"What if you get married?" I said only half kidding.

"I'll never get married mom." Then we snuggled in and their warm bodies comforted me for the moment. But after they were asleep, my disease began and my mind and heart started racing. I would crawl into my closet and feel surrounded and safe by the smell of cardboard paper and confined space. There I would slowly fall asleep; keeping the door opened a crack. I was more afraid of being locked in than the fear of my kids waking up. I would listen to the gentle sound of their breathing and clutching my boxes would fall asleep too. In the morning I would wake up before them and try to be a proper mother until it became too much and I had to again escape into my closet. I always left my children in the care of my eldest daughter Elena while I hid, and they sometimes thought of her as a second mother. When I got really desperate, I let my mother babysit.

The most off the wall experience in my boxes happened in my walk- in living room closet in Hawaii. I am deathly afraid of rodents and after a time away from Hawaii on one of my runaway trips, I found the house was overrun with mice. I called a well known nationwide extermination company and they sent a guy to my house named Kirk. He was very young and I had a bad vibe about him as he did his inspection of my house. He seemed very young, inexperienced and didn't communicate well. I called the company where I was assured that he had been working many years and was one of their best technicians. As usual I believed a man who pressured me and didn't trust my own feelings. I let Kirk return to my house many times because he had found an entry point in the stove that had to be blocked.

One day, I was in my boxes in the closet and a mouse came out to say hi, I freaked and called Kirk. When he came, he methodically took out all my boxes from the closet and I was in there with him for an hour helping. When he found the mouse at last, I screamed and he smirked. He grabbed it and unexpectedly took his large shoe off and stomped the poor mouse to death in front of me. I screamed again and he smiled and gave the weirdest laugh. I had never seen this man even smile before.

Two months later, Kirk Langford was arrested for the murder of a Japanese visitor, Masumi Watanabe. He would be convicted of her murder and sentenced to life. They never found her body but he confessed to throwing her dead body in the ocean. His story was that he was in the area working when he encountered Masumi on her daily walk. He said the sun was in his eyes and he hit her with his truck. Although she was slightly injured, he convinced her to go inside his truck, and in fact someone saw a dazed Japanese girl getting into the passenger side of the truck from the driver side. In the truck, he asserted that she started freaking out, not understanding what he was saying as she didn't speak English or why he couldn't find her house and after breaking the windshield, managed to open the door and fell out at a high speed. He said she hit her head on a rock and was not breathing and that he feared he would lose his $70,000 a year job because he had accidents before and had been warned if anything else happened he would be fired. He then put her in the back of his truck and continued on his daily work schedules. He stopped for plastic bags and tape and after work tried to bury her in a bag. My daughter always says people in Hawaii are up in your business, and proving this, a homeless man saw him digging a hole, and took down his license plate. He then went to another spot where he threw her in the ocean like discarded garbage. At sentencing it was discovered that he had killed cats, attacked another Japanese visitor and was accused by his wife of domestic abuse. I was locked in the closet with a convicted murderer and possible rapist. But more importantly, I had awareness of something being wrong and I didn't assert myself yet again. The boxes lost their appeal after that.

This whole incident brought back my attack at nineteen and now I was even afraid of my closet. I grieved for Masumi and her parents who came from Japan to hear the last hours of their daughter's life from my ex exterminator testimony. I thought of the small detail of police finding her broken glasses in his work truck.

He was a liar, and I was a liar for not acknowledging my own trauma and hiding from myself the truth of what I had been through. It was then, that the closet or my boxes couldn't pull me out of the anxiety and depression that ruled my life. Panic attacks started happening in the closet or in the house which I rarely left. I even woke up from deep sleep with a pounding heart sure of impending disaster. I was not even safe from attack in my closet. I was as misplaced and messed up as the boxes.

My closet time had caused me to become oblivious to life. As the years piled on, I couldn't see what was happening in front of my eyes. One of my daughters was a lesbian and I found a diary of someone talking about a girl in their class who was ignoring her and her pain of not belonging and I truly didn't know it was my own daughter calling for help. Who is this troubled girl I thought and how did this journal get in my closet?

I was truly the last to know everything that occurred in my house. While the world turned, I was the proverbial camel with its head in the sand or in my case; a box. In the end, I ended up living with my ex husband a meth user and dealer and even though there were glass pipes all over the house he had designed and made himself, I didn't connect it with drugs until my ten year old son informed me of his addiction.

The neighbors thought I was on drugs because I lived with him, a well known, except to me, drug dealer. "She never leaves the house, she must look like hell," they told my neighbor. My oldest son was showing signs of severe mental illness and my youngest daughter was dating a convicted rapist. I had cement stuck to the bottom of my feet and couldn't leave the house or deal with the reality of my life. I knew it was time to get help and start thinking outside of the box, but how?

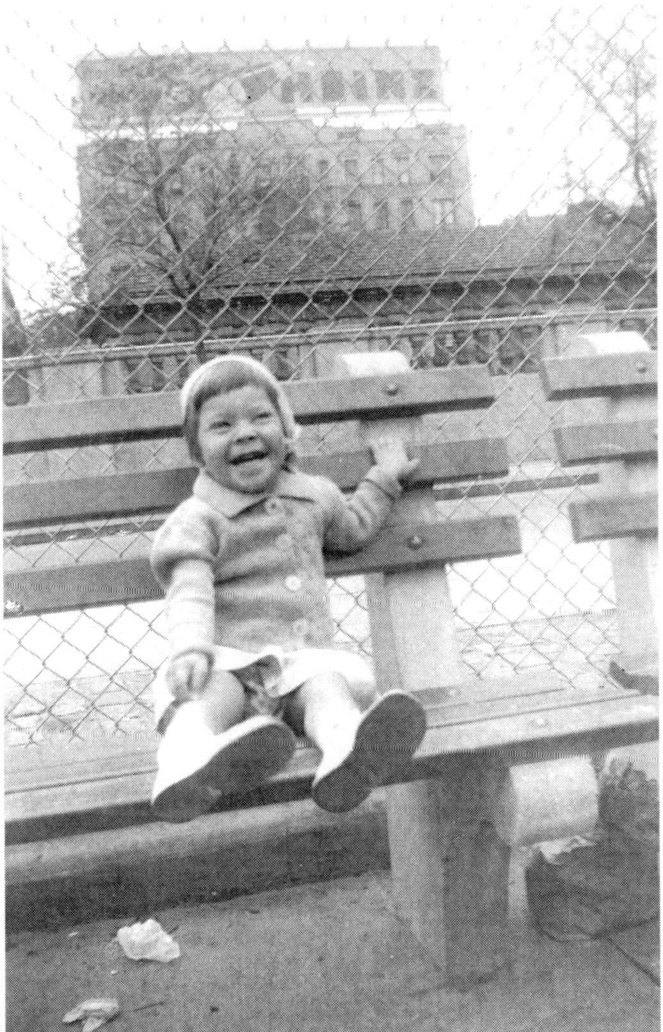

CHAPTER 26

Smiling Prohibited

My mother forbade me to smile in photos after I started school. I was confused because when I was small she always said I had an amazing smile.

"You smiled in that class photo," my mother is yelling. "I told you not to smile when you take a picture, you look meshugana (crazy person) when you smile." Since, I was an obedient child, I'm looking at the myriad of photos of me looking like the sad star I put on the board under the happy sun to encourage good behavior in my own students. It was strange, because everyone else also admired my wide smile but like most things she liked, she eventually and inexplicably rejected.

The day before she died I was at the epic play "Le Miserable" on Broadway. This was my fifth time experiencing Jean Val Jean's misery but the first time my own took precedence. Tears splashed down the tent of a dress that was supposed to hide my flab from my mother.

I didn't want to go to New York fat. I was in the middle of my boxes with major drama from my daughter Junette's determination to screw up her life with a former police officer on trial for raping a teenager in his police car, a crack head ex- husband I was living with out of financial desperation and panic attacks so severe, I was unaware of any of the other above events. All this showed in my body which at five one and 193 pounds had me living in the most beautiful island in the world- Kauai, doubting my ability to go on living.

"Your mother is asking for you." My aunt Sylvia called me. My mother was in a Jewish care home in Brooklyn since she had broken her hip and now though rehabilitated, my father had refused to let her come back home. He had Parkinson's disease and my mother's mental illness had drained him despite the respite from his mistresses. It wasn't that he didn't love my mother in his way, but he couldn't take my mother's tantrums anymore. Who could?

I called the home and my mother almost unrecognizable as a meek lamb said, "I thought you were mad at me."

"I could never be mad at you mommy," I said, meaning it. "I 'm just busy with my kids and stuff." Liar I thought.

"Could you come and see me?" she asked. She never before had asked for me. My heart thudded as I wondered how I would be able to take the trip and worse, let her see me like this. She took my weight issues personally and would berate me for "letting myself go."

I bought the most slimming black dress I could find, and somehow boarded the plane. When I got there, she was showing me how she was healed and could walk, and go home but in a moment she cried that daddy didn't want her back.

"I love you Marilyn," she said, "I'm so glad you're here." She never said that.

She never mentioned my weight, seeming not even to notice.

I was there a week and pleaded with the projects to move my parents into a ground floor apartment, one of the care home's stipulations of her coming home, talked to social workers and begged and finally persuaded my father to let her come back. I told her this when we visited her.

"I can't take it anymore here," she said. Her bed was so small and she shared her room with a woman who had Alzheimer's disease.

"I'll get you out, mom, daddy promised to take you back. Please be patient. We can take anything if we know it has an end date."

She looked me and said, "How did you get so wise?" She never said that either.

The next day we got a phone call. It was my mother. She also never called.

"They gave me a cup of hot chocolate this morning, and it's so delicious. I had a wonderful dream last night."

"That's great mom," I said, so relieved I was finally helping her. That night the care home called us.

"Your mother attacked her roommate and was moved to the psychiatric ward at Staten Island Hospital."

"But she was doing so well, and I almost had her back home."

Then I remembered her telling me; I'm only good when I'm sick. My real self is kind of mean, and that's a good thing for me.

It was hard for us to get to Staten Island but my father arranged a car service to take us that day. The steel door had multiple locks. When I saw my mother she looked ten years older and her sparse hair was plastered around her head. She had wild eyes.

"I have to take the trolley, but I don't have five cents. Please give me the five cents. Carl, where are you," lucid when she eyed my father.

"Why'd you do it?" he asked.

"She was doing disgusting things to herself and I thought it would be better here but they make me go to meetings and won't let me sleep. I'm too old for this."

Then she was out of it again. I felt isolated and scared like I did at Prospect Park so long ago but stepped in front of her and said,

"Mommy?"

She looked at me, focused and lit up.

"Marilyn with the smiling face. I love you honey"

"I love you too mommy."

I hugged her but stepped back when she got angry.

"Where's that damn nurse? I have to go to the bathroom."

I was crying so hard that the nurses had to hold me up as she returned to her childhood.

"Daddy, give me money for candy."

Her voice had a whining sound. I was collapsing on the nurses as they comforted me. I was careful that she didn't see me.

"I have to go to the bathroom. C'mon, c'mon."

She looked at one of the nurses and smiled a toothless grin back at us and said, "We had a fight, but we made up."

I talked to the social worker and they promised me they would put her on a medical ward that night because she had a kidney infection, so again I went to bed hopeful that I could save her.

That morning I was awakened by ancient wailing. My father, with his advancing Parkinson's disease could hardly speak by then, so I thought I was dreaming for some minutes. When I slowly opened the door he was pounding his chest.

"She's dead, your mother is dead."

"It's not true. You're lying."

I knew the force that was my mother couldn't just leave like that. He's insane I thought, finally losing it, after taking care of my mother for so long.

I called the hospital and a doctor was immediately put on, a bad sign in my experiences with the medical profession.

"Your mother was put in the regular ward last night and died peacefully in her sleep."

"It's impossible. My mother was getting better. Someone killed her. Or she is still there alive and you can't see it. She's pretending. She's good at that." I really believed this with all my heart.

The doctor's voice took on the voice of someone speaking to a mentally challenged person. "No dear, she's gone. Her organs just gave out."

"No," I said. "Please she wouldn't die like that. She was coming home and out of the psych ward. That's what she begged for. Why would she die the same day she got what she wanted."

I stopped, realizing clearly that she planned all of this. Again my mother's mental illness proved too much for me.

She asked for me to come so she could see me before she went. I was there for only two weeks. She knew my father was taking her back reluctantly. She couldn't handle rejection. She loved him so much. He didn't want her anymore. She had planned to see me before she decided to die. But I still wasn't sure she was dead.

I knew that I would have to make all the arrangements and I knew it had to be a Jewish burial. It was December 7th and a Friday. My father and I went to the funeral parlor that handled my older aunt's funeral and with my mother's money that had not gone for the restaurant for my father, had not gone for clothes for her, or a house we begged for, we paid the funeral director. He called a rabbi that was willing to do the service before sundown and I called my eldest daughter who was closest to my mother and she flew in from Minnesota. My mother would be buried in New Jersey where she was born.

The next day at the tent that had been set up for the service, I took the director aside and asked. "Is everything alright?" I really meant was she really dead but he misunderstood.

"Don't worry, everything is taken care of." I wanted to ask if he saw my mother's body, but I was too ashamed.

The rabbi was young and he took me aside and gave a graveside service that was quick but moving. I held my daughter and her slim body trembled in my arms. Could I conquer my fears for her? The rabbi took me aside afterwards and talked to me.

"You have to go back to your roots for you mother's sake."

I didn't deserve roots.

Mommy always said I married beneath me. Didn't she realize there was no beneath? I was the worm under the bottom of the barrel. My roots were in that coffin, my larger than life mother. I couldn't save her. I couldn't save anyone, my daughter, my panic attacks or my obesity. The rabbi was kind, but he didn't know this.

"Thank you," I said, and he gave me and my daughter a torn black cloth to pin on our clothes, symbolizing the tearing of garments that symbolizes deep sorrow.

Then we left her alone, driving off in the limo. I had nothing to say to my father, his mistress or my crying daughter; so as we traveled to Brooklyn I chatted with the limo driver about anything but what had just happened. We then went to a Chinese restaurant where I almost choked on pork spare ribs.

Back home, I took a small bench from my mother's room and went to my old room where I covered the window and sat for three days and wouldn't come out. I tore my clothes and scratched my arms in a lonely form of "Sitting Shiva," Jewish mourning.

In most Jewish families, the rabbi and guests come and keep you company while you reminisce about your lost loved one. But I was alone. No one was there for my mother. She had pushed everyone away. So I sat alone, praying, fasting and writing poetry to her, realizing I had lost the only one who had ever loved me, however rough the love. My father called me to eat rice and beans but for once my insatiable appetite was gone.

Later, I looked at other photos of me as a child. In one, I am in a stroller leaning to one side with my hand reaching out and a panicked look on my face. I am not crying. I peer again at the miserable look on my face, I remember. Mommy is taking my picture but I can't touch her. I am too far away and terrified.

"Pick me up, Mommy, don't leave me alone."

After the funeral, I am in my mother's bed and can smell the mixture of her face cream and mustiness. I focus on her polyester pants suits hanging in the closet and finally, the tears come.

I scream, “Come back. I’ll be good... I’ll never smile again.” That was December 7th 1995, and I kept that promise for more than five years.

CHAPTER 27

SEND IN THE CLOWNS

When I was four, my father took me to a rare outing to Steeplechase Park in Coney Island. At the entrance was the midway was called the "Pavilion of fun." Waiting for me there was a clown with what looked like a flashlight. He grinned and pointed the flashlight at me and as a whoosh sounded, my dress flew up. I was standing under a blow hole but the clown had tricked me into thinking he had power. As I tried in vain to pull down my dress while simultaneously clinging to my father and screaming, I vowed never to trust a clown again. I also hated the Jack- in- the box toy my father bought me at the park. When you turned the handle a song began and with the line "Pop goes the weasel," another mean clown popped up to scare me. I think of that clown now as a misogynist dressed in sheep's clothing. So, with my history of not trusting my instincts and marrying anyone with a pulse, it is not surprising that my third husband was both a clown and a pedophile.

Manny was so besotted with me, that when we met at a restaurant bar, he forced a gold necklace on my neck that weighed a ton. I refused to accept it and he refused to take it back. He later sold it for thirty dollars to get drugs.

He came into my life after I came out of the hospital and was just newly pronounced sane. I think they were mistaken. At least that is my excuse for marrying him. He was like the character in the Kung fu movies he was addicted to, who makes the hero laugh at his comic antics; a survivor. He acted the buffoon to hide his true character and a person has to be smart to do that. I needed a good laugh and financial support, so I sold out and started seeing a man I didn't love or was attracted to. He wore the “mask of sanity” as many sociopaths do but inside lurked a criminal mind. He wasn’t a good person just a very good actor. He lied to me from the beginning, telling me he was divorced and had one child. He was married and had five children in the Philippines.

Manny was a talented mechanic who also had a talent for making money but never keeping any of it. He gambled and drank and used the promise of money or fixing cars for blackmail. He had a third grade education, but he once built a tow truck without a blue print and could tell what was wrong with any car by starting the engine. Manny was good at entertaining us with stories about his life in the Philippines when it was under Martial Law and even more dangerous than it is now.

He had been a boxer in Cebu, and had never lost a fight. Even then, at thirty eight, though short in stature, he had a thick neck and muscles that reminded me of Popeye. He opened jars and pulled carts with his teeth until they fell out from the meth he became addicted to. He spoke Pidgin English and had a flair for comedy and entertained us with stories which can’t be retold properly without his gravely voice and wild gestures.

He would take off his shirt and show us a big scar. You know how I get this? My kids said, “How?” their mouths wide open.

“Hon, (he always called me Hon) I was in a village away from my family and I was gambling my paycheck and winning, when bad men accused me of cheating. They stabbed me, put me in a sack with a big rock and threw me in the river. I’m good like Houdini kind man, and I untied myself and opened the bag. I good swimmer hon. I born near river. I swam back to village. Next day, I got one bolo knife and saw the men and they ran away screaming, ‘Ghost, Ghost.’”

Another story he told was about a cow. "I punched a cow dead, because he ate the garden I planted for my family. I was boxer before, oh I just went up to him and punched him plenty times. He dead now." My kids said, "But uncle Manny, the poor cow." He said, "Life in Philippines, hat wok (difficult) my kids had to kau kau (eat) so cow had for maki."

The last story is not one he told my children; why he left his family and came to the United States. His parents had been born in Hawaii, but his mother and father both married to other people had run away to the Philippines together and he was the product of that adulterous union. One day, he overheard his nephew (who he had invited to stay with him) tell his wife to meet him under the mango tree at 11 at night. He had been away for weeks working and gambling and his young nephew and his wife had gotten close, too close. He took his bolo knife (most of his stories had a bolo knife in them) and waited in the bushes. "They were there making love against the mango tree, my mango tree so I waited until the right time, when they were going to "cum" and ambushed them waving my knife and screaming 'Hah, Hah', they were so scared, they ran naked in the bushes and didn't come out all night. I wasn't going to really kill them, just scare them but I couldn't stay in Philippines after that.

A baby was born that his wife named Manny Junior and eventually the nephew moved to the US and they let bygones be bygones. The wife found someone else, and I unluckily found Manny.

But seeing Manny in his dramatic moments was fun for the kids. They asked, "Uncle Manny who is our president?"

"George Washington," he said as they fell to the ground cracking up. They told him he was wrong. "It's Ronald Reagan," and he made them laugh harder by mispronouncing it like the clown he was. But inside the clown lurked a predator, an addict, and a sociopath. He made my children happy by taking them out to restaurants and buying them toys. He gave them money to scratch his back but his humor was a tool. He used it to get what he wanted and let others slip up thinking he was stupid. He finally got a divorce because he was also a sex addict and at the time I was studying with Jehovah's Witnesses. He bought me an engagement ring and pressured me to have sex with him. Although he wasn't my type, I will admit he taught me more about pleasing a man sexually than anyone else. It was all about him. But by the time we got married, I knew he was a pleasure pig whose slop would be drugs and guns.

He also had a monstrous temper and once pulled down an armoire that weighed more than he did because he thought my son had stolen his cell phone. He was wrong. My daughter had taken it to college. He became out of control when his marijuana or money went missing. He never blamed or hit me but living with a person with no boundaries was scary and I was always waiting for the other shoe to drop. Once he ran out in the street when he thought the same son had stolen his pig's head. He fell to the ground and screamed and kicked like a two year old. "I'm hungry, I want my meat."

I was the one that threw it out because it looked and smelled disgusting but was too scared to admit it and my son and his wife who had just moved in just laughed, not knowing the extent of Manny's tantrums and addictions.

He was more dramatic than jealous, but I remember that when I discreetly told him his friend was hitting on me in a club he stopped traffic by blocking the exit of the club with his truck and started screaming, "I'll drink your blood Rafael." He never seemed to get arrested for this. I think the cops enjoyed his performances.

One day, after being married to him for a few years, I went into the empty room adjacent to my teenage daughter's bedroom and noticed holes drilled into the wall. I couldn't figure out how they got there, dumb ass that I was, so I called my best friend Doni. She clued me in that they were peepholes and Manny was a voyeur that was perhaps molesting my daughter and I should try to catch him in the act. That night I slipped out of bed when he thought I was asleep and tiptoed downstairs. I slowly opened the door to him naked and masturbating while peeping at my sleeping daughter. I felt sick to my stomach. Not wanting to alarm my daughter I pulled his ears really hard, and said, "Get out."

He left but I am guilty of letting him back when my daughter's assurance he never touched her coincided with our electric getting turned off. He promised never to do it again, but Doni armed my daughter with a squirt gun with soap to defend herself and told her to dress in the bathroom until the wall was fixed. I watched him like a hawk and did some investigating. Others had noticed his lust for my daughter and his friends told me he admitted being in love with her. I started hating him and myself. He paid for her graduation party like a love sick puppy and he half moved out. Yet as time went on I knew I had to be strong and leave. I couldn't forget the good that Manny did for me and stayed with him until the there was a sign that was too big to ignore, even for me.

One night after a few weeks absence, he came home drunk and unloaded a gun on the kitchen table. I started planning my escape. I made my reservations for a flight to Minnesota where I had just been notified I received a scholarship to finish my BA. The same day, I discovered I was pregnant with Manny's child.

PART 5

THE OPEN DOOR

"I TORE MYSELF AWAY FROM THE SAFE COMFORT OF CERTAINTIES THROUGH MY LOVE FOR TRUTH; AND TRUTH REWARDED ME"
SIMONE DE BEAUVOIR

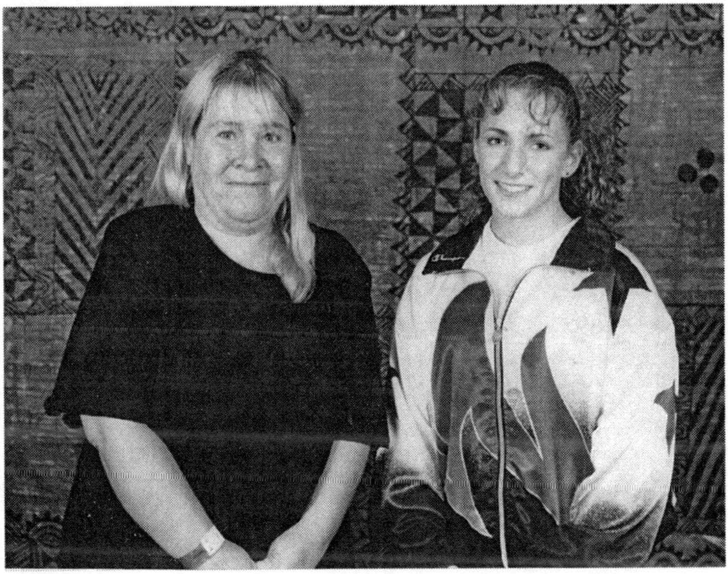

CHAPTER 28

Shannon Miller and Me

I love the Olympics, especially gymnastics. It never matters how overweight I was, I always see myself as an athletic just a smidgen away from the physique of an Olympian. My daughter's were also gymnastic fans and in my self-enforced stay at home years, watching the Olympics became a family tradition and gymnastics in particular, our family bonding time. I would go into my fantasy world and be my favorite gymnast. That changed every four years. I was Olga, Nadia and Mary Lou. I would be tumbling along with the competitor even feeling her heart beating as we both leaped in the air or balanced on the four foot width of beam.

So when I had the chance to see our favorite Olympian gold winner, Shannon Miller at the Hawaiian Gymnastics Classics on February 22, 1997, I forced myself out of the house. Amy Chow, Amanda Borden and Jaycie Phelps were also being featured as exhibition performers but we loved Shannon Miller the best. She had this "tude" that we respected and also it was funny how she raised her arms and "smiled" when she was about to perform. She was someone to reckon with and when they won in Sydney, I celebrated by inviting people over to my house. No one came. Now I could see them in person if I could only get myself out of the house. I made that my goal and went a bit further out of the closet every day for two months.

I walked very slowly out of the house my heart beating like a bird's wing against a glass window. I ended up in the emergency room with a panic attack but did that deter me? No siree. I even wore my hospital bracelet from my trip to the ER.

Junette, my youngest daughter was away for her first year of college and I was determined to see her look of amazement when she saw a picture of Shannon Miller in a picture with "Moi."

After their flawless performance, I went in line and paid my seven dollars. She was very gracious and smiled her performer smile, but I was shy and nervous. I crossed my hands in front of me. I didn't want to accidently touch and defile her; then I smiled. Me and Shannon Miller wow!

Wow is right when I saw the photo. At almost 200 pounds I felt like I would be sick when I saw myself next to the Olympic athlete

Doni, my best friend, laughed and said, "You look happy." Happy is not the word I would use. That photo is not only a reminder of what damage I had done to my body by eating myself to a near heart attack but also why I couldn't face the world. "I'm hideous," I said over and over until I got to the safety of my home. The year before, getting my daughter ready for college, I was told if I didn't stop obsessing over Junette's escapades and take care of myself, I would end up with a heart attack. My panic attacks increased as my weight did and though I had returned to my own house in Honolulu and she was safely in college, I still had not dealt with my past and didn't want to. But the picture, it haunted my dreams and I knew I would have to show it to my daughter when she came back on summer break. She came back a mature young woman who had turned her life around so much she was featured in the local paper, "The Garden Isle" in a local bad girl does good, article. She laughed at the photo while I cried and then she left. Now it was my turn to change my life around and I decided to start with my binge eating.

I knew I had an eating problem for a long time, but I was not diagnosed until I moved my family to Minnesota to get my college degree. I was applying for a grant to get into a famous eating disorder clinic and it went like this. You know you have an eating disorder if when asked to list your prior diets, you ask for extra paper. I was accepted, but the grant fell through at the last minute. I wasn't ready to stop binging anyway. But while in Minnesota I found out about the Jenny Craig program and decided to ask my mother for a loan.

"Feast or famine," she yelled over the phone. "Do it yourself, you don't need any Jenny to tell you what to eat. Push yourself away from the table".

The table was the least of my problems. I ate everywhere and everything. I wasn't choosy, but I had my favorite binges; potato chips, ice-cream, ravioli and any and all carbs. I saved my pennies to join Jenny Craig. It sounded so rich, so private for someone to focus just on me.

I lost 8 pounds the first six days and forty pound in four months. The nine hundred calorie was so easy for me to follow that I pronounced myself cured. I thought I had found my nirvana and at 136 pounds I quit without going on the maintenance phase of the diet. Of course, I gained it all back and more because the root of my food addiction was not addressed. I eventually lost seventy pounds but that would be later and I used the new and improved Jenny Craig program not as a crutch, but a tool to go along with the holistic plan that would change my life. I am almost on maintenance now but it never would have worked in the long term if I hadn't faced the reason behind my self-hatred and need to punish my body with excess food.

Now, I look at the photo of me and Shannon Miller with compassion and respect. I don't hate the woman in the black dress next to the woman in the red, white and blue. I am sixty years old, and ready to jump on the parallel bars and walk the full length of the balance beam without falling.

CHAPTER 29

THE OPEN DOOR

It was the day after the Millennium and I found myself in East Harlem at my sister Carol's house. I had not slept yet and when I looked at my reflection in the mirror I saw an unhappy, bloated, face looking back at me. I was uncomfortable in my body and possessed a terrified, unstable mind. The night before had found me squashed on the couch next to my late father's morbidly obese ex- mistress, who made me at almost 200 pound look almost like a lightweight. She hated me and I hated her right back. Wilma was an alcoholic, uneducated, Jew hater whose German parents had convinced her that Hitler was well meaning and The Holocaust never happened. She never missed an opportunity to insult me or point out my flaws on the rare occasions our paths crossed. When she looked at me she saw my mother. My mother had been used as an excuse for my father never having to leave his wife for his many mistresses.

"How can I leave her, she's sick," he would tell them when the truth was more devious and complicated. He had a crooked loyalty to his only legitimate wife. To him, my mother was his responsibility. He couldn't understand her, the voracious reader who forced him into libraries and drug stores to get her fixes. But he knew she loved him more than life and helped him in ways that Wilma never could or even imagine. My mother took my father out of the kitchen where he chopped and prepped for French chefs who treated him like the garbage they made him throw out. She helped him apply to be a porter for the city where he eventually became the king of the projects. How my father could marry a teetotaler, an intelligent daughter of religious Jewish parents and have a German Nazi lover who according to my father wouldn't leave a party until the last drop of rum was consumed, I'll never understand. I can only surmise to my father, pussy had no barriers. He eventually dumped her when he got older and tired of the constant partying. Many other women would take her place.

That night I was at a party with my sister Carol, Wilma's daughter. She always came to my defense as her mother insulted, chided or berated me. The bottles of rum at the table were disappearing at a fast rate, as the Latin music kept the loneliness in that room invisible to all except the one person there that wasn't drinking,

That night, Wilma had taunted me by shouting, "You can't dance," and this hit me below the belt, if I could have found one that fit me, because not only was my mom a talented dancer and met my dad at a Latin dance, but I had danced Salsa on stage.

Bristling with rage, I dragged my cumbersome body on the floor to dance as mean a Mambo as my weight allowed.

"Oh, so you can dance," she unhappily commented. I unhappily rejoined her on the couch breathing heavily and knowing she had won by having me stoop to her level.

Back at my sister's house, the blaring televisions, including my nephew's who had an obsession with advanced electronics brought me to my knees. He had the latest stereo system with the largest speakers I have ever seen or heard which brought the movie "The Matrix" so vividly into my tired brain. I thought for a minute I was not only in a theatre but in the movie itself.

I was laying in my sister's king sized bed along with five female relatives who were in various stages of inebriation. The snoring competed with the TV, but the winner was my niece Allegra's hobby; fighting on chat lines.

Allegra was a tough New York street wise Latina with a heart of gold as bright as her huge hoop earrings and Minnie Mouse tats, but her shouting, "I axed the fuckin chronic bitch to challenge me," challenged me to pray for death.

Carol couldn't sleep with the TV off and I couldn't sleep with it on, so when the ruckus quieted down a few decibels, I got up and went to the bathroom. It was eight a.m., January 1, 2000, and I was fifty years old. I was overcome by what seemed like a lifetime off loneliness and the certainty I didn't belong anywhere but home. I desperately wanted to be there with the covers forever pulled over my head. I tried to cry but couldn't. This time I didn't wait for the familiar sadness to turn into despair, depression and panic. In that cold East Harlem morning something amazing happened, a revelation. I felt a glimmer of hope, growing into an insight that started to seep into my being. It seemed to come not from the depths of desperation but somewhere light and almost spiritual. I knew somehow, I would find a way to recover from this profound pain that ruled my life. Who knew a book from a spiritual Toltec master from an ancient city outside Mexico would lead me out of this mess? But that's what "The Four Agreements" would do.

CHAPTER 30

Standing on the Threshold

It was now 2006, and I was passionately reading books and practicing my new tools of healing. I started with The Dalai Lama because he was serene and cried in front of people unashamedly. Now, I was working His Holiness' first of the 3Rs, which is respect for self. The second is respect for others, and the third is responsibility for your actions... Respect for self is first, because the other two are impossible to conquer without self respect. I actually thought I respected myself and was respectful to other people but on closer inspection, I realized I had no idea what truth or self respect was. I abused my body, eating like I was a garbage disposal, not even tasting or liking half of what I ate. I stayed with men who cheated on me and abused me physically and mentally. My children sometimes also joined in calling me "tree trunk thighs" or "bag lady." I was filled with so much fear and hatred. I not only allowed this treatment but thought I deserved it.

I was always the feverish pleaser and the more I slaved for this impossible feat, the more my self hatred increased. I couldn't be perfect so when I inevitably screwed up, I felt even more worthless. When I succeeded in some goal, I felt depressed.

At my college graduation at the age of thirty eight, my accomplishment so amazed me, I cried throughout the ceremony. From the start when a trio of classical musicians played until they called my name and handed me my diploma, I was filled with an emotion I thought was self respect and pride. But, afterwards at the small graduation party that my good buddy Sally Perez had made for me at her house, I started feeling almost suicidal. I thought it was the green dress that was a size sixteen, or the fact my eldest son wasn't there because of his severe schizophrenia and depression. Photo after photo was snapped as the self hatred grew. I felt lonely and ugly, there with my small group of friends and family. I looked in the mirror that faced the dining room and my image repulsed me. I was fat and hideous with a crooked imbecile like smile and a crossed eye. I hated myself with a fervor that frightened me. I had worked so hard and had been so excited before the graduation. What had happened?

I now know that when something good happens to me, I get depressed afterwards. I had invited my parents to my graduation and they sent me a card, my mother too ill to attend, my father too disinterested. Education wasn't a value to him. I wanted them to be there and for once to be proud of me and prove I wasn't the worthless piece of shit I knew I was. But even if some miracle had happened and my mother would have shown up, she would have rained on my parade. I heard her voice that day. "How did you let yourself get so fat? Why didn't you win the award you told me you were up for? How wasteful to buy a cap and gown at your age?" I had heard that all before at my Junior High School graduation. Although I knew this intellectually, my fantasy fueled my self hatred and shame.

I carried a tape of my mother's voice and no matter how I tried I couldn't shake the self-contempt that made me sabotage myself. Therapists told me I had a great deal of self awareness. Self-awareness didn't change my mother's tapes melded inside of me. I later would do something like keep my pen in the ready position, which my ex boyfriend hated and when I noticed, the self hatred built up so loud I couldn't silence it. "Stupid, you need to be punished for this," and I couldn't stop myself from poking myself with the tip of the pen like he did before my rational mind took over.

Or I would lose my glasses for the umpteenth time and hear my mother's voice. "Careless Marilyn, you would lose your head if it weren't attached to your shoulders." I detested myself with a hatred that seemed relentless.

In Nathanael Brandon's book, "The Psychology of Self-esteem," he speaks about "respect for truth versus rejection of the truth."

I had rejected the truth because I was told not to dwell on bad memories and thought I had succeeded with my "remarkable" self- awareness. But I fooled myself as well as others by half truths and total repression of other truths. I had suppressed anger and redirected it to myself. I had let men, bosses and teachers abuse me because I thought I deserved it. I had disrespected the events in my life and like a Pandora's Box that was half open; the poison was escaping into my bloodstream. I knew that day, I needed to release that poison by facing and respecting the truth so I could face and respect myself. I couldn't be healed unless I released the secrets that shamed and almost destroyed me. Self- respect would begin by telling the truth, but where was it? It was too late to turn back. I was already in and above my head.

CHAPTER 31

WORKING IT OUT

It was morning and I had just arrived at my job at the YWCA when I heard an unearthly scream. The staff congregated at the door of Sandy, a resident, who started shouting, "She's dead, she's dead!" As far as I knew Sandy didn't have a current roommate because the last one had left because she never took a bath and collected garbage. Her room, a tornado of thrift shop clothes piled high on her bed felt like the back room of hell. We all stood outside the door, the fear of death, though unspoken blazed on our faces. As the police and ambulance arrived I learned that the dead woman had checked in the night before high on drugs, and playing "Iron Maiden." When Sandy threatened to call the front desk, she said, "Fuck you" and passed out. When the newcomer could not be awakened for the free breakfast and her sleeping position seemed awkward, Sandy realized the woman was dead. The nameless woman had died of an apparent drug overdose during the night. Sandy fell over the crowded room screaming and broke her ankle.

For day's afterwards the residents requested the room be blessed and cleansed by a Hawaiian priest. Priscilla, the manager was trying to deal with that and all the other crisis that come up when you are dealing with women in various stages of chaos.

I was the AmeriCorps volunteer and I had a small office in the back near the unused pool. The Fernhurst YWCA was once an elegant house that watched over young ladies of decent backgrounds while they went to school or worked in Honolulu. Now it was the dumping ground for women whose lives for one reason or another had taken a turn for the worse.

The Y had three tiers of social status. On the ground floor were the women with children, and other abuse victims. Some elderly, thrown away mothers and heart patients took up the rest of the first floor. On the second floor, were the usually heavily medicated mentally ill and drug addicts with an occasional prostitute thrown in. This was the problem floor. The third floor held the so called elite- Asian students, and the elderly regulars who were snowbirds from Canada or Minnesota. Somehow, the women on other floors never complained that the upper floors were bigger or had better showers. They preferred staying with women of a similar persuasion.

What all the women had in common was a kind of homelessness that put them in vulnerable situations. The Asian students needed the thirty five dollar rate which included three adequate but terrible meals, the tourists found some kind of family in a place they had frequented in a more elegant time and the others, well the others were just in survival mode.

During my time there, all residents on every floor requested my services one time or another. The Asian students who were English challenged and culture shocked, found in me a friendly tutor, when a term paper crisis loomed in a language that seemed inhuman. The most vulnerable women came in with problems too large for me or anyone to solve but most of the time, just needed to be listened to. I filled out forms for housing, I called social agencies that would help them with the myriad of problems I was confronted with and sometimes I even hooked them up with jobs through the agencies the Y was connected with, or the internet.

Miki was one of the regulars who came in to use the computer program that designs cards she would never send to anyone. She escaped an abusive marriage in New Jersey and she and her daughter who lived in

Hawaii had been evicted by a landlord who was turning paradise into even more of a parking lot. She was always very cheerful yet distant. She was on social security and did not want any of the services I offered to her. She had many acquaintances, but no close friends and preferred it that way. Her cheery demeanor fooled me at first, and I tried to befriend her, she said "Marilyn, I don't want to hurt you but life with my husband was such hell, I prefer to live the rest of it unbothered by people, so please let me do my own thing here." I recognized then, that I put on the same false cheerfulness.

Rosa was an elderly mixed Hawaiian woman waiting for elderly housing. She had been wealthy at one time and tried to keep up the façade, with her manicured nails and faded silk shawls. The other women gossiped that she was an alcoholic. I believed them when I helped her fill out an elderly housing application and smelled the fumes as she leaned toward me.

Filling out applications is my specialty. I have been filling them out since my first job application for the co- op program at my high school William Cullen Bryant in Long Island City, New York. I had been deemed to be an underachiever, really undereducated from a slum, to the ritzy school where, I was not able to keep up in the academic course. There were three programs: the academic, for those bound for college, the commercial, for secretaries and the general, for the sweat hogs, the underachievers. My mother ordered me to enter the cooperative program where I would go to school one week and work one week at the Metropolitan Life insurance company. The consequence for this was I would be in classes that were suited for slow learners and would get the general diploma. I balked at first not wanting that last row in the last seat, but my mother really needed the sixty two dollars every two weeks and I had failed the first two programs. I went to the interview with my gloves and hat on like proper young ladies were required to in the sixties. I see myself in my minds eye in my suit nervously filling out my first work application. Somehow with the pen in hand I felt a fleeting moment of confidence. I had to pass an IQ test which I did well in and a typing test which I barely passed. I was so happy when the interviewer told me I was hired. This was my first real job at fifteen and I was offered either the typing or file clerk position. I chose the file clerk at one dollar a week less, because I thought it would be less stressful and my typing skills were minimal. My mother had typed 90 words a minute on a manual typewriter but I was not interested in anything she was good at.

I started working at the grand building at One Madison Avenue. I felt so grown up taking the train to work and eating lunch in the free cafeteria. I was allowed to keep a few dollars a week for my train fare and a few extras. My first paycheck I bought a set of knives. It felt so chic walking in Lord and Taylor's buying a set of steak knives. And I half kidded, if all failed I could use it to kill myself. When the week of work was over and I was just getting sick of filing, I was back at Bryant High School with the dummies as the Co-op kids were called. I was finally the smartest kid in the class and that confused me. I was called smarty pants and it reminded me of first grade when I got the lollipops or being the best reader and yelled at for "not using the classroom neatly." Soon, school became boring, and work tedious. I was fifteen and already stuck in a rut. I helped everyone in our class fill out applications. It seemed so hard for them and so easy for me. I thought it was a fluke. I didn't know then that filling out applications was a skill I would use to help people navigate the system of poverty which would become all too prevalent in my life.

Now I was queen of helping other people at the YWCA, and it was déjà vu all over again. I filled out applications and helped until my head hurt.

Vicky was a young girl with narcolepsy. She would instantly fall asleep and hit her head on the computer. I would hear a bang and there she was snoring. I was supposed to leave her alone and not wake her up, but the thud when her head hit the table brought on panic and I dreaded her appearance at my door. She disappeared one day. The residents never stayed long.

Alicia was the obese prostitute who needed money for her not so hidden crack habit, and Lou, was the butch lesbian out of jail that would try to bully me into breaking the rules of computer time allowance. I was scared of her, not because she was a lesbian but she had muscles and tattoos and could kick my ass. I cringed when she came in and became the bullied child yet again. Thankfully she wasn't that interested in computers or getting a job so she left me alone.

Clara was a woman of fifty who had been a college professor, but obesity and diabetes had forced her to quit before getting a pension and she walked with a cane. She was very smart but naïve about the poverty system and I found her senior housing and disability again by filling out the application she had never heard of. I started hanging out at various public social services and being part of governing boards. I learned what I had already known. Poverty is a full time job. But I helped one woman at a time and in the process I started seeing myself in a different light, a competent light.

I did go on to college after having children and realized I was not an underachiever. In my thirties, I received a college degree and started working as a victim advocate for my internship at college. My professors at college became my mentors convincing me that I was smart enough to graduate. I minored in criminal justice and began seeing what horror humans inflict on each other. I had to attend criminal trials until my panic attacks returned with a vengeance.

Now, I was again starting over as a volunteer and by being enmeshed in other peoples' problems I learned that by treating people with dignity I was gaining dignity for myself. By respecting and acknowledging these women, I was respecting and acknowledging myself. By listening to their stories, I would be able to clarify my own story. So, I filled out application after application.

The day of the cleansing, I greeted the Hawaiian Kahuna with aloha. I followed him and Priscilla, the Y's director who was sweating and flustered. She was a good Catholic and couldn't understand what the fuss was about. We went from room to room listening to Hawaiian prayers and watching the Priest wave a cedar like branch around. I felt unexpectedly, calm and free of anxiety. This place, this job, had done for me what nothing else up to this point had, a sense of place and inner peace. By nurturing, I was being nurtured. By being helpful, I had helped myself much more. Other people's problems were more than a distraction from panic. It led to the beginning of my healing.

CHAPTER 32

Master Class

After the Millennium, I took up reading again. Like my mother, I used books my whole life to distract me, to disappear into a dream world that held no pain. But like a bandage on a gaping wound the pain and infection festered underneath.

But this time, instead of mysteries, travel guides or erotica to soothe me, I read not to escape but to confront my demons and find answers to my illness. Anything that was positive, spiritual or healing leaped into my hands. But I was tired, so tired. I had no emotions. I didn't feel anger or love or even lust. I didn't know who to be angry at or who to trust. If I did have a fleeting emotion, I was too afraid to express it. I was beat down literally and figuratively and life was getting old.

Yet, I had this seed of hope, which I couldn't let go of, and it was about to germinate into a tree of life. I just didn't know it yet. One night I found myself on my knees with praying hands.

Surprised, I found myself in tears, praying, "Dear Lord, help me, I put myself in your hands. I will do whatever it takes to heal. I don't deserve you but I love YOU."

"Please forgive my sins which are many and I love You, wherever you are."

Not being a religious person, I was skeptical at what had come out of my mouth. But that night I slept soundly for the first time in years and I woke up with hope. Lightening hadn't struck, but I felt less anxious, more at peace. I read later that the Dalai Lama had said that sleep is the best meditation. I know now praying helps too.

In one of the books I read a traveler in Tibet in the 70's had given a Tibetan man a photo of the Dalai Lama as a memento. The Tibetan man had fallen to his knees in tears because the spiritual leader he worshipped, but never laid eyes on was now an image in front of his eyes. I didn't know anything about the Dalai Lama at that time but such devotion intrigued me.

I read about the Dalai Lama and the calmness he presented, but the first real healing came in the form of an Australian woman on my break- up board on the internet.

She was tired of hearing about my broken heart and abuse and directed me to a book **"THE FOUR AGREEMENTS"** by Don Miguel Ruiz, a Toltec Master. He talks about the Toltec's being an ancient people in Mexico who were called **"women and men of knowledge", and states: "they were scientists and artists who formed a society to explore and conserve the spiritual knowledge and practices of the elders."** The Toltec is not considered a religion but a way of life that embraces happiness and love.

The first agreement is to "Be impeccable with your word." I read it and realized most of my problems had to do with not telling the truth. On page 28 he says, "Every human is a magician, and we can either put a spell on someone with our word or we can release someone from a spell." He tells the story of a little girl, one like me who liked to sing, but her mother in a bad mood tells her to stop and that her voice was ugly. "But the daughter believed what her mother said and in that moment she made an agreement with herself. After that she no longer sang, because she believed her voice was ugly and would bother anyone who heard it." And later on page 35 "Whenever we hear an opinion and believe it, we make an agreement and it becomes part of our belief system. This little girl grew up, and even though she had a beautiful voice, she never sang again. She developed a whole complex from

one spell. This spell was cast upon her by the one who loved her most; her mother. Her mother didn't notice what she did with her word. She didn't notice she used black magic and put a spell on her daughter. She didn't know the power of her word... and therefore she isn't to blame. She did what her own mother, father and others had done to her in many ways. They misused the word."

Genius! I had been living under a black magic spell placed upon me by my mother's mental illness. I had the power to break that spell. Just like Dorothy in the Wizard of Oz, who held the power to go home, but didn't realize it until the end of the story. I could break the black magic spell of my agoraphobia and panic and it didn't matter if my mother was to blame or if she really loved me.

I would begin by making a new agreement. The agreement I made that day was to live as if I were already healed, as if I already knew what truth was. I was good, I was powerful and I would be impeccable with the truth. The problem was I didn't know the truth yet, but no matter, I would learn.

I threw out all my junk food and called AmeriCorps (The Peace Corps for America) for an interview and also returned to therapy. This time, however, I called a local sex abuse line and asked for a female counselor trained in rape. I moved like a robot, like someone was guiding me. Could it be some spiritual master of ancient times or even THE Creator? It would take every bit of strength and many miss-steps to rid myself of the buried anger and horror of my life, but I felt determined and hopeful. Like the cowardly lion in the Wizard of Oz, I discovered I already had courage but hadn't known it until now.

PART 6

BY ALL MEANS

"VICTORY BELONGS TO THE MOST PERSEVERING"
-NAPOLEON BONAPARTE

CHAPTER 33

DAMN, I SLAM

I walk into the dark cavern of a room signing up for the Thursday night poetry slam. There are a few teenagers in baggy pants in a group practicing their lines with hands punctuating the air, a microphone and me. Ok, I showed up early. I have to take the bus home. Holy crud, the stage is ten feet tall. I'm sweating. I never sweat. I fell off a stage while dancing in Spain, I can't do this. No, not the poetry, I mean climbing up on that stage.

I am third on the roster; I sign my name as Maya from Makaha so everyone will know I live on the west side 30 miles away. The seats are empty so I rationalize no one will notice if I crawl up the stage, humiliate myself and go home on the bus. As usual life has other plans for me.

I wait, and the room starts filling up, and I mean filling up like a club on a Saturday night. The mistress of ceremonies comes up to the mic and slams some prose that brings on a familiar terror that I am not good enough to compete with anyone in any area, and more importantly how the hell am I going to climb over all those people sitting in front of that huge stage like disciples at the feet of Jesus. The major players here are the organizers and regulars who seem very comfortable on that high stage. I start to enjoy the slamming but as names are called up, I notice being third on the list in no way makes me third on the stage. I start to feel like this is some kind of "in group" and how I feel about groups is well documented. It is getting late and I am still not called. I run into the bar, and throw back a glass of wine and even though I don't drink alcohol, don't even get a buzz. No one speaks to me and yes, I am the oldest person here. As the slam continues, I notice with relief, not everyone is good. Some are excruciatingly bad and as the end nears and I am not called. I push my way to the front of the crowd and tell the DJ's helper, a kid of sixteen, "I have to go home. I have a curfew, so call me already."

He relays the message to Master Kimo and I ask for help from him to pull me on the stage feeling a bit bad as most have leaped up without a thought. "Here's Maya from Makaha," he shouts. I am scared at first, not used to being in front of an audience anymore, but the girl who went before me went over the allotted fifteen minutes and ranted on and on about perverted men, incest, and rape. Maybe, I think the crowd will be ready for an old broad with humor. There is a prize of one hundred dollars for the winner which I suspect is not going to be me but a selected group holds up cards from five to ten like in the Olympics for gymnastics. I am out of my element I think, though I don't have an element.

I take a deep breath and say "Hey guys, I'm a teacher so if any of my students are here, this is not me." I start with a poem about my mother, very tame very passionate, but memorized and since most of the youngsters have pages obstructing their faces, this is already different. I use my theatre voice, loud and clear and the murmuring turns into total silence, as even the crowd of drinkers in the back stop to listen. Then I start slamming, forgetting my injured aging dancing body and do what even the major speakers had not done. I belly dance, I salsa, I project, I'm alive!

"For all you ladies who have been mislead and mistreated, and all people who have been hurt and bleeding. I stand here naked for you to see. Who's on top?"

Who's on top now?

You made me drop down

Kneel with confusion

Not an illusion

You disregarded basic decency

Treatment without leniency

I kill you with kindness

Sweetness drips blindness

So sickening yet it's fitting

I'll make you do my bidding

What do I need from you?

I have to think that through

Who's on top now?

You almost made me drown

Can't make you love me

But feel my energy

And give me your fake support

That always fall's short

Of keeping me afloat

Yet…

What will I want tomorrow?

Not your heart, it's hollow

Not your friendship

You lying hypocrite

Or your salty kiss

And your quick dismiss

Who's on top now?

You'll be the one to bow

Do ya think I'll still care?

When you disappear

I just kept you around

So I could feel the sound

Of evil going down

What happens to the souls that lose their minds?
And then are forgotten by humankind?

There's no Bedlam for them to go;
Only shopping carts in piles of snow

They're destined to wander in a daze
Hiding from the sun's punishing gaze

Muttering phrases that make no sense
Unless you understand the brains defense

Occasionally exploding with dangerous results
Stabbing innocent adults who wrote

Open the doors of locked up places
Thrown into a sea of scary faces

Demons inside; no place to hide
If they don't behave; they're thrown aside

Sanity is tenuous without a hand
I once belonged to that sad band

Please keep them safe; for all our sakes
One in four will face their fate

I stop, and then without any paper, I turn back, "This is for my mother"

Don't send me flowers, you always said
Bring me purple flowers in their bloom
You were not easy
You were a proud rose with a thorn that stung many who attempted to enter your inner sanctum
But I will fill a room with lilacs!
Because your being shines like remembered rain
And the lavender fragrance of your soul engulfs me
Yes, lilacs for mother and my love

Stunned silence, then applause and I revert to the older woman who has to be helped down the stage by a teenager. No matter, I am in my element after all. I get nines. I leave quickly because the fear is back, and at the bus stop the familiar depression after achievement returns with a vengeance.

The next day I get calls from people who had been there, mostly college students who were friends of Nanise, my daughter's roommate at Earlham College in Indiana. I was pronounced "bad" which of course means I'm good. I'm also exhausted. The strain of leaving my nest of safety to climb a mountain of hope is too hard for me right now. I decide to slam in front of my screen until the stages get lower or I feel higher.

CHAPTER 34

A DATE WITH AGORAPHOBIA

It is 10 a.m. and I am getting ready to go on a date. My date is coming to pick me up at 6 p.m. but no matter. There is already a sinking sensation in the pit of my stomach. Dresses and lingerie are strewn about as agoraphobia and fear of rejection surface like a recurring nightmare.

Since my hair is sparse and as limp as thin spaghetti, my preparation is turning into perspiration. My friends call it my four hour hairdo. I laugh, but inside I call it my four hour ordeal. First I wash it with any shampoo that promises to turn the skinniest hair into a glorious crowning glory. I want to believe this is true and have spent a lot of money on these evil promises. After the shampoo, I put on the conditioner which is supposed to strengthen and thicken limp locks. I keep this on for an hour hoping against hope to gain more hair. Then, I blow dry my hair upside down, a proven method to increase density or get dizzy. I can't say after all this that I look that much different, as my crowning glory is less than royal.

Of course there is a shower, where I shave any offending hair that might sprout from places almost illegal in Western society. Then I take a bath in almost boiling water with herbs that will eliminate any odor that might detect me as a human being.

Then it is time to put on my face. I get all my makeup from my eldest daughter; leftovers for free. I spend time trying to hide the acne scars and wrinkles that are Mother Nature's final joke against me. Since I rarely wear makeup anymore and my memory has diminished with age, this process takes an eternity. I have to remember not to pile on the foundation like I did in my teens, when I was trying to hide the worst case of acne, maybe on the planet.

I am getting tired by this time. I am old and nervous, not a good combination for a good date. But it is a ritual I seem possessed by. I still have to perfume my body with Jennifer Lopez's "Live" to feel less than dead, and to find a dress that is alluring yet, conservative enough not to spell, "one night stand, or even worse; old hooker."

I wish I could be like a woman I saw at the bus stop who had one long thick hair sprouting from her chin like a weed. My first thought was that she didn't own a mirror, but after a chat realized, she was just happy in her skin and accepted her appearance, even liked the hair, naming it Leilani the second. I wish I could be like that but my vanity doesn't want to give up the fight for almost pretty just yet.

The bell rings and my gentleman caller stands at my doorstep with one dying rose in a plastic vase; how sweet, how kind, how oily. He is also vain because I notice he combs his few hairs from back to front, making it hard for me to suppress a nervous giggle. I am not the only one it seems that has hair issues. Why do men think we will not know they are bald? Hey, how do they know I am not balding?

This particular buffoon, and the men I date are mostly buffoons, is a lawyer. I somehow can't imagine him in front of a jury presenting his case. Whatever he says will be somehow overshadowed by his stunning appearance.

"Your house is green," he says, stating the obvious.

"It's not green," I say, it's "Ocean." I have to say this to some visitors who are stunned by the sea green walls. "It's comforting and relaxing."

"It's too green, your painter should be taken out and shot," he replies, handing me a bottle of a California wine that promises stimulating conversation, or yuck, more.

"Thanks," I say.

We leave in his red Porsche, a staple for aging barristers. I suddenly feel tired and stupid for preparing for this loser. We have an uneventful dinner at Outback Steak House, even though I had told him I rarely ate meat. I am grilled more than the rare meat I choke down.

"I don't usually date woman as old as you are but I will make an exception in your case," he says. There is zero chemistry and he is a blithering idiot. I am repulsed, so in inverse order of a date's desirably, I inexplicably become the talkative social worker, the hostess, the cheerleader on crack. I massage his aging ego, until it flies upward like a wayward balloon, I so hate to dump someone. Some men get what I am up to, most don't. I am exhausted by the time the date ends and as he drops me off at my door, I am reminded of my mother's favorite saying, "Was this trip necessary ...?"

I got tangled up in the World Wide Web by joining a dating service that promised more than any could deliver. I went on many "date zero's" which means, first dates with men I "talked" to on the internet. They were zeros in many other ways too.

Dating at fifty is as bad as it sounds. I was married most of my life and all this was new to me. With agoraphobia, getting ready for a date with a stranger changes the word I used to use at fourteen, which was "exciting," into "torture" which usually extended to the dates themselves. I decided in the beginning to date one hundred guys, but it all went wrong when I got to number thirty four.

Number thirty four's handle was shy808. After talking to him for a few weeks, I knew shyness was only one of his issues. Ok, he told me he had other issues. He stalled about meeting me saying he had been depressed and dateless since he got laid off. I should have not gone there, but he was cute, at least in the tiny photo he sent and had lived on a kibbutz and was cute. Ok, I said that. We agreed to meet and have dinner at Chili's. He was to pick me up at home. When I saw his shiny black truck pull in my driveway, I was still putting on my earrings with shaking hands.

The phone rang. It was him. "I can't do it," he says.

"Do what?" I said.

"Come in," he says.

"Whatcha talking about, whatya mean?" I always revert to my native tongue, Brooklynese when confused. Now, I know a red flag when I see it, but you have to understand the extent of my frenzy in getting ready. I wasn't going to let this one get away so easy.

"Get in," I barked.

After twenty minutes of using all my social work and mothering skills he agreed to come in. He walked in, a hulk of a man, with huge "deer caught in the headlights eyes." Before I could adjust my idea of his size to his photos, he ran to my back wall sticking to it like what we call in Hawaii "one opihi" (a clam that sticks to the coral reefs of Hawaii).

"I can't commit, I can't commit."

"Commit to what?" I asked quietly (my anxiety always turns into calmness in the face of insanity) "Does, this mean we're not going to Chili's Restaurant?"

"I can't commit to Chili's," he kept on repeating.

"Can't commit to Chili's?" I almost asked, but he was already running, getting into his truck and hitting the metal so fast he hit my aluminum fence when he backed out of my driveway. That's it, I thought, I'm done with dating. I stop here!

Since I was eight and left with my grandmother, I always calmed myself; acting or dancing in front of dark

TV screens. There, I had complete control of the outcomes of my drama unlike the real world. I became adept at adopting alter egos who had more confidence than I did.

Around this time, in front of the screen, I had been developing a new persona, Magic Maya. Maya is a name with many meanings. In Hebrew "Mayim" means water. I always loved water, from bubble baths to the blue-green salty oceans of the Pacific. Then I found out that Maya means dream or illusion in Hindu, taken from the original Sanskrit. I knew then I would add Maya to my name: Illusion or not. I would stop dating losers, stop being afraid and honor my life and change the illusion into a good dream.

While I was dating men who were bad, not in a good way, my prose started slamming in a bad way which is good. I practiced in front of that dark screen and felt ready for my close up. That is, if I didn't have to leave my house to do it. It would take every ounce of courage to perform at a poetry slam for kids like me; fifteen and over.

CHAPTER 35

THE HYPNOTIST'S FISH TANK

"This is not going to work."
I am in the plush office of a medical hypnotherapist. It doesn't feel like a carnival or a party where I will bark for biscuits or perform other parlor tricks. Dr Cullen walks in, a scholarly man in a turtleneck sweater and black slacks. He appears almost comatose himself; he must have majored in New Age at Sedona University.

This is not my first time attempting alternative methods to deal with my mental illness. In 1972, I was part of a medical trial hypnotherapy program at Maimomonides hospital in Brooklyn, where they were testing pain free childbirth through hypnosis. I went a few times but the doctor said I was holding in burdens I was not ready to release. Those burdens included an eight pound baby that also didn't want to be released. I think I was in a trance when they had me walking around to X-Ray every few minutes to see if I needed a Cesarean section in the 48 hours of labor. They finally knocked me out and tried to pry him out.
I woke up and said, "Where's my baby?" and they said, "Still inside."
I said, "Oh no you didn't" in my best Brooklynese and they knocked me out again. Finally my baby was born and I learned two things: Doctors can be crappy; you can handle more than you think; anxiety or not and hypnotism doesn't work. Still, I was in my new mindset of trying everything to unlock my secrets and anxiety.

My new female therapist didn't agree with my new experiment. She warned me that bringing back the rape too fast or carelessly might be unsafe. I had every right to believe her because she specialized in sexual abuse, but I was annoyed that she stopped me short of telling my story. I was in a hurry to tell and get well. I knew I had garbage inside that needed to be released. I had flashbacks of horror; something elusive was nagging me. Would finding the truth set me free from fear? Burying the shit stank. I was ready to release the demons that were interfering with my life and continue my healing regime.

The doctor's soothing voice was so over the top, I almost giggled. But he seemed sincere and I was eager, so when he directed my attention to the aquarium in the corner of the room, I got serious. I had noticed the large fish tank, who wouldn't? It took up half the room, but I hadn't realized what a big part it would play in the following scene.

The lights were lowered and I was directed to concentrate on the fish and slow my breathing. It wasn't hard to do because I had always been fascinated by fish. Fish are fascinating, and when the silence continued a memory flashed through my head.

Hiroki, my last boyfriend had a fish tank, and when I moved in I looked at the fish. They were grey and plain looking. He told me they were old and when his children were young they fished them out from a nearby stream. One day when I first moved in, I was mesmerized by the largest fish I had named Oscar. That morning, Oscar who was eleven years old was acting weird, if a fish could act weird. Hiroki, who was obsessively cleaning as usual didn't pay any attention to me paying attention to the fish. Oscar was trying to move a huge rock in the tank. He struggled with the rock pushing and struggling with it. I wondered why, but I just accepted the behavior as fish frolic. The next day Oscar was dead in the tank. Hiroki was upset, and said it was a bad sign in our budding relationship, but I was wondering why Oscar had wanted that rock moved. I philosophized that he wanted to accomplish something magnificent before his death. I did too, but my life goal was always centered on a man. I was so desperate to find love I stubbornly accepted abuse in my relationships, even if I had to move rocks to get it. All the fish would eventually die during our sick relationship. They were old, after all, but I remembered Oscar as I watched the tropical fish in schools of vibrant colors moving with their own tribes, not wanting to get involved with fish of a different color.

I came back to the present hearing the therapist voice asking me mundane questions in the getting to know me process, and I told him some of my trauma but I felt relaxed and content to speak while watching fish.

Then he said, "Marilyn do you remember the rape?"

"Which rape? I've been raped more than once."

"Tell me about it," he said.

The last rape was Sabola, who was called Sab for short. I looked it up later and it means pepper in Egyptian. Sab was a math professor from the Big Island, the largest island in Hawaii. I was given his number by my neighbor who had met him at the hospital where her husband was being treated for a brain tumor. Sab had cancer too, and was well known in his community as a compassionate teacher who took in students with family problems. She showed me a newspaper article about him. Good credentials surely. He picked me up in a rented Mercedes Benz, as middle aged and suntanned as a California movie director. This would be a first date and we would go out to dinner at a famous Honolulu hotel.

He had a strange way of mixing intellectual conversation with "My last girlfriend had multiple orgasms" on the way there. He also confided he was separated from his Egyptian wife and teenage son who had Juvenile diabetes. He was Turkish he said, but born in Egypt.

"See, I am white under this tan."

"Who cares?"

I just looked at his large nose and eyes that moved as fast as his tongue.

"I come to Honolulu twice a month for treatment, and we can be good friends," he said with a meaningful look.

After a quiet dinner where I knew we had no common ground to base a friendship on and no chemistry for anything deeper. I refused an after dinner drink at the hotel bar.

"C'mon just one drink," he said as we were walking around the plush hotel and stopped in the main corridor of elevators.

"The bar is on the rooftop," he said pressing the button of the elevator.

"No," I said, and he held me with one hand while pressing the elevator door which had come down empty.

I fought him screaming, "No."

For God's sake where were the people? This was a popular hotel. He pushed me in and I screamed kicking and fighting, not believing this was happening to me again.

When we got to his floor, I laid down on the hall carpet yelling, hoping someone would come out of their door or something anything. He pulled me by my hair inside the room.

He was breathing like a pit bull in heat. "You American Jewish bitch," he snarled, his mask unveiled. Stupid, why did I tell him my mother was Jewish?

I am Egyptian and I hate Jews.

"You told me you were Turkish," I said trying to calm him.

"I said I was born in Turkey, you whore, and you act just like my first American girlfriend who broke up with me after she took my virginity. So innocent, so unaware of how dirty she was. I'm married and live with my Egyptian wife and son, but she has advanced diabetes and can't handle my sexual power. I don't want to fuck her anyway, she's too fat. My son is sick from this country. I would never leave him for any American Jewess whore like you. I hate Americans especially ones like you, so blonde, so friendly, and so uninformed about the world situation your people started. Just want to be happy," he spat.

He threw me on the bed and I knew I would fight this time even if I lost my life. I fought like my Chinese astrological sign –the tiger, punching and kicking him. He had cancer, he had to give up sooner or later.

He didn't bother to take my clothes off; he just ripped my panties off. He was huge and I couldn't fight the hate that made him a superman. He held my hands in a vise like grip over my head and then I realized he was experienced at hurting women. I didn't stop resisting. The pain was blinding but this time I would go down fighting.

Afterwards breathing heavily, he said, "I know I'm not a good lover because men with huge penises don't have to be."

"Make love," I said my mouth dry and sore. "You call raping me love?"

"Of course I didn't rape you." He was calm with dead eyes, "How can you say that? I'll take you home."

"No, I said, call the police," but he was leading me into the bathroom and washing the blood off of my face.

"You're a nice girl." Where did I hear that before? I doubted my sanity but he drove me home, smiling at our neighbor. She came over before I could slam the door.

"That's the kind of guy you should date, clean cut," she said giving me the thumbs up. I locked my door and took a bath rushing to get his smell of sweat, chemicals and hate off of me.

He called me constantly trying to convince me not to press charges or call the police. He begged me.

"I have cancer, I'm dying, and my wife would die."

"Let her die too," I said, not meaning it. "I really don't hate Jews. My doctor is Jewish."

"I hope he kills you."

"I'll lose my job and my position in the community if you spread these lies about me."

I kept his number under my bed for years with his name and school imprinted on my brain. Why was I always tricked? Why did I trust that people were basically good? What about me was so deserving of punishment? These were the questions I asked the ceiling as my soul cried out for a cure. Would all my secrets have to be extracted by a hypnotists spell?

"You will remember all we talked about and feel calm until next week."

But even an upbeat suggestion couldn't stop my pounding heart.

I realized why confession in the Catholic religion is so vital. Revealing my sins and shame felt right. My burden was a snake shedding his skin. My shame and self hatred that contributed to my self imposed imprisonment was being lifted to the sky little by little. In a dream, I saw the beauty of telling. The hypnotist was the priest and I was paying for release, sort of like the "indulgences" that Martin Luther had protested against so long ago. Like a priest caught in the act of having sex in the middle ages, I had been hung in a cage and made to starve to death. My cage being my closet where I binged, dieted, and held on to my deserved punishment; my indulgences' were granted when I wasn't killed by my attackers or told my secrets. I was learning that keeping those secrets was the real sin.

As we got closer to the original rape, I would start suddenly in panic but the hypnotist took his time and I was able to trust him and the fish. The shame of the things I had caused and allowed didn't have to be suppressed any longer. I felt like a cloud lifting higher and higher with each visit and freer between visits. My friends and therapists were skeptical but I am nothing if not stubborn. I continued until all the truth poured out and like a samurai warrior, I destroyed the poison of my secrets. Ever hopeful or naïve I prayed to be rewarded by the beauty and peace of this truth.

My only apprehension was that my mind harbored a monstrous secret that might affect my often tenuous grip on sanity. The hint of this was the agoraphobia which like a lingering cough prevented my healing. Would I find the secret key to unlock the door of my torment? I would have to look at a lot of fish to find out.

CHAPTER 36

BY ALL MEANS

The best complement I ever received was from a Japanese man I met online. He pronounced me a magician. I was singing at the top of my lungs in his hotel room, "Beautiful, beautiful, beautiful truth, don't leave because I can't see you."

Hideki had never heard of the Scottish group "The Proclaimers," having lived in a small village in Japan's northern prefecture Hokkaido, and stared at me like I had three heads however mesmerizing, a bit other worldly. He was the head speaker of a conference of quasi religious/self-development cult. They were conventioneers at the Hyatt Regency Hotel. We met for a drink at the pool bar after heating up the internet with discussions about cross cultural communication, travel and social responsibility. There was no romance, but the passion of our talks led me to as unusual a world of peace, cross cultural communication and lasting friendship. Of world communication, travel and social debates heating up the computer from Japan where he lived with his wife and two grown daughters. We decided to meet to continue our discourse in person.

We moved from the pool bar to the hotel lobby. I had requested this because when the wind blows crazy in Hawaii, my hair blows in a very unattractive way into my sticky lip gloss. Yes, I was overdressed in a red geometric wide skirted dancing dress. I could blame this on my Latina heritage where overdressing and over accessorizing is de rigueur. But the truth is my fear of rejection is so huge when I meet anyone for the first time, I always resort to overdressing and lip gloss. I did resist the J-Lo hoops, but at the last minute feeling underdressed I put on a pair of chandelier earrings which contrasted sharply with the shorts and sandals of the hotel tourists.

We made quite a stir in the lobby as the staff and convention goers alike stared at the overdressed white woman and the Japanese tourist. I heard whispered, "Old prostitute bothering a Japanese guest," in a stage whisper by the front desk personnel. I also heard, "Couldn't possibly be a couple," by passing guests.

I am always the last to know I am making a scene, always happy to have arrived anywhere.

The Japanese side stares were probably what prompted "Is it possible to go to my room to continue the conversation."

I hesitated only a minute as I looked at this short fifty year old man with horn rimmed glasses. He had a spark of intelligence and goodness that leaped out at me. Trusting my instincts was new to me, but I decided to again take a chance and we went up to his room.

Taking chances was something I was taught was not acceptable as a child. I was going to end up in Brooklyn, a secretary married to a Jewish man unlike my mother who now said she knew better. Taking chances only caused punishment, control and unhappiness. But I saw the opposite at home. My mother who had the fortune of five thousand dollars kept it in the bank and refused to relinquish it and my father had the fun without it I learned.

I took many foolish chances, not learning as a child the difference between opportunity and danger. I embarked on many journey's and found many men who would marry me, thinking by doing this I would avoid the many catastrophic proclamations my mother had made regarding my future. This backfired on me as my agoraphobia and panic held me in a tight grip until I decided to use my brain and imagination that had lifted me from poverty to freedom.

So, I find myself in this hotel room and after a few awkward moments while I sat stiffly in the high back hotel chair and Hideki, my friend rustled through his bag to show off his photos. In my experience the Japanese attitude toward picture taking borders on the holy. If you don't have a picture to prove it, you were never there.

We started talking about music and I told him about my failed Broadway career and before you can say Karaoke, we were singing. We went through his repertoire which consisted of Swanee River, Yellow Submarine and a final rendition of Amazing Grace, where at the end he had tears in his eyes and I had joy in my heart. Who would have thought it? I told him about my failed Flamenco dance career and then he started singing Granada where I did an impromptu Spanish dance. That is when he called me a magician.

I was happy. Maybe magic is as good a remedy as any other for healing.

My name is Edith, but I was called skinny by my brother. I was born in Englewood New Jersey. In the Jewish religion we are named after deceased relatives and mine was a great aunt. My mother's name was Lena Jaffee. She was born in Russia. She was a good mother always cleaning and cooking. She loved us very much and tried her best. My father was born in Poland. I called him Pa. He had two jobs. We didn't get along but the older I got the more I realized how good he was. I thought he was cheap when I was young.

I was brought up in Williamsburg Brooklyn and years ago it was safe and clean. It sure has changed. We were five children living in three rooms. My mother kept the place immaculate. She was a perfectionist.

My responsibility was just to do good at school. I think she wanted us to get a good education and get an office job and not have to work in a sweat shop like she did. My special place was my bedroom, just kidding. It was the library and my closet.

PART 7 ZEN

"AND NOW MESSIUR ET MESDAMES, SAID POIROT RAPIDLY, UNDERSTAND THIS; I MEAN TO ARRIVE AT THE TRUTH. THE TRUTH, HOWEVER UGLY IN ITSELF IS ALWAYS CURIOUS AND BEAUTIFUL TO SEEKERS AFTER IT"
THE MURDER OF ROGER ACROYD
AGATHA CHRISTIE

Jan 18,

I have to go to a good hospital where I can get shock treatments. I can't kill my husband with my behavior. What happened to me? I can't live like this. I am worse my mind is gone. I don't want to be mistreated. I never harmed anyone. Please be good to me. Have pity on me. I hope I can behave myself. I need self control. I didn't wet my hair for 2 days or pour hot soup on my head. I am losing my hair. I look terrible. I aged 10 years. I always looked younger than my age. Now I look older. If I felt better I wouldn't care. I need my privacy. I love my home. It is a lovely apartment. My room is so large. But I want to feel better. Please have pity on me. I'm a human being. I want to be treated like a person in spite of my looks. In the hospital people judged me by my looks. If a person is not nice looking people are cruel. I am not that way. People laughed at me. I want humane treatment.

Today is Martin Luther King's birthday. What a great man he was. Dr. King up in heaven, say a prayer for my recovery. I always loved you and John and Robert Kennedy. The country lost 3 great men. I think I'm going to shampoo my hair in cold water.

CHAPTER 37

FATAL ERROR, OPERATION ABORTED

The next week finds me again lying on the hypnotherapists' couch. I am getting too comfortable with the fish, the voice, and the leather. He tries another method to entrance me as I'm beginning to call it. I try not to laugh as he takes out a pendant with a hippie psychedelic design. Is he going to swing it in front of my eyes droning, "You are getting sleepy?" But he only tells me to concentrate on the pattern. I see his serious face looming above the pendant and perceive a telepathic movie screen. Did I go under? It must be true. I am mesmerized under his spell, I have never felt so relaxed, wait, is he saying that? I am there but not there. Flashes of visions, dreams and unwanted reality appear in my minds eye, I hear him but the flashing pictures are impossible to turn off. His voice seems to become stronger, louder, and I feel less comfortable but still unable to move or slow down the action.

Then, my senses are fully awake, enveloped in an odor, what is that smell? I see lights and an operating room. Oh, I relax for a minute. It's ether. I must be having my first baby, but no, this is not right. I see a male doctor and my first daughter. Elena was delivered by a woman near Chinatown New York by a Chinese woman doctor. I gave birth "au natural" in the labor room with a young Chinese girl whimpering next to me.

This doctor is also Asian but he is a Japanese man and I am terrified. Is that the rape flashing on the screen in my mind, or something even worse? I try to get off the couch but I'm paralyzed. I see my mouth moving so I must be talking but my brain is on the screen. Gone is the operating room. I hear music, louder and louder and I feel a strain in my throat from trying to be heard above the Latin Jazz. His name is Carlos and he says he is Puerto Rican, but I am thinking, liar. One knows ones own. He has a weak mouth and few words, not my type. He's telling me I'm beautiful. They all do when they want sex or love. He just wasn't right, I didn't trust myself but I knew I didn't want to go in a car with him. But again, wasn't I always wrong? Didn't most people say so? I had only blamed Linda, because I was afraid of blaming men. They would leave me, and the hideous monster I carried inside of me would be seen by others.

But the secret that is about to come out is not the rape at all, but also a despicable secret. I'm despicable. I treated a rapist like a king so I could survive. I did that at nineteen. I came out of it with a few superficial cuts but the inner cuts were much deeper. I never reported the rape. I am guilty of letting another woman perhaps not survive in Carlos' car. Guilty, Guilty!

I am sweating and am back again to that hospital operating room and with tears pouring down my face I remember why I was there. I was having an abortion but it is not from the rape. I am older and have all my children.

I was convinced when I sat in the social worker's officer in the hospital. I won't have a monster's child, and she agreed, but the father wasn't the rapist at all. I never got pregnant from Carlos. This was Manny's child; and he had been a kind of monster, lusting after my daughter and bringing weapons to my house. I had to leave my home because of him. I had no guilt at the time; anxiety was about the surgical procedure, not the morality of it. But the day of the abortion I had a nosebleed so severe, I called to cancel, but they said the operating room was ready and I had promised to be there. I always keep my promises, no matter how hard, mommy had taught me that. I wake up in the recovery room, with a nurse pulling my hair really hard. "Wake up already," she said.

"Don't cry, you weren't crying when you got yourself pregnant." I wanted to scream at her, punch her, stab her, but just like the rape, I was silent. Inside, however, I had a feeling of loss. It was over. Or was it?

A week later, I am superficially healed but frantic calls from my doctor every hour left me strangely calm. "You must return to the hospital at once."

Was it all a big mistake? Was I never pregnant? The doctor was upset, and he explained to me, that it didn't work.

Huh?

"The baby is still there, alive and even growing despite the abortion."

I didn't understand.

"How could this be?" I answer slowly, "Maybe we should leave it like this. The baby wants to live. I don't want to go through that again."

The doctor is livid. "It's impossible; you will have an imbecile, a damaged child." My self esteem is no match for his education and position of authority.

"You can't have this baby", he said sternly. It will be a burden for your children, your husband, and most of all your mental health. How can you bring a possibly severely disabled child into this world on purpose? How can you deal with it with your mental illness?"

He kept phoning and pressuring me. Having another male's domination was like a second assault. Now, I know he was afraid of a lawsuit, but then that thought never occurred to me. I again let a man, a doctor, this time intimidate me. After the second "procedure," I developed pelvic inflammatory disease and had to be hospitalized. Certainly the doctor wouldn't make the second mistake twice. He said I couldn't have any more children, but the moral impact of what I had done reached my heart. This was a reasonable punishment. I started having nightmares of children without limbs and monsters who looked like rapists and murderers who looked like me.

One day soon after this, I went home and fell to the floor in despair. I called to the heavens and petitioned a million prayers, lit a candle for that baby who wanted to be born, and cried a million tears. I prayed for forgiveness and I wasn't even religious, but I couldn't forgive myself and the memory hid in the deep recesses of my brain only to come out on that couch. I thought I had mourned for the child who wanted to be born, but then erased the incident from my conscious memory. It had been buried deep inside and kept me inside. Depressed and angry, my anger was not at the rapist, the doctor, or even Manny who had encouraged the abortion. I left Manny soon after that but he wasn't capable of guilt so he never understood my pain.

When I was ten, I accidently killed my mother's pet bird. She had let it out of the cage in the kitchen without telling me and I opened my bedroom door. Whack!

"Murderer," she screamed at me as I cried and cried.

Now, I still heard her sing song voice. "Marilyn Is a worthless human being, a killer. The bird was more important to me than you."

She later said she was sorry but her words became my tape. Although she never knew my crime, I would conduct the punishment; self- imprisonment. I had eaten myself into oblivion and locked myself away from humanity. I was not worthy of being around others, was not worthy of being angry at anyone. I knew that, though not exactly why. Anger was for good people, and I had made sure if not consciously, to surround myself with other violent abusers. I wanted to be punished for my crimes.

I knew somehow it was time for forgiveness that day at the office, I invited in peace and truth. To remember was important. I will never forget my child who fought to be born or my part in his demise. But, I would try to forgive myself.

The hypnotherapist wakes me up gently with a suggestion, "You will look truth in the face with courage and wisdom. Open your eyes and remember." His sad eyes looked at me, and he asked how I felt. "Light," I said, very light."

CHAPTER 38

Zen

Not so long ago, I met a man named Dave that looked great on paper but after dating him a month, I had a funny feeling about him. Something just wasn't right. I used to ignore red flags even if they slapped me in the face but now I trust myself and did the unthinkable; I told him I felt uncomfortable in his presence and couldn't see him anymore.

"You're an ugly old bag anyway," he said, confirming that my gut instincts were correct.

I laughed in his face.

My new therapist didn't rush me to confront the rape; instead we concentrated on changing my habit of agoraphobia with new habits that were akin to flying from a trapeze without a net.

"Do whatever it takes to go to work. Make a new habit of getting out," she says. It's not easy. It's hell to suffer a million deaths just to be able to work. It's doesn't get easier but it gets to be a habit. I act "as if" I am well, and three years ago I accepted a job as a teacher even though I have to commute on the bus to do it.

"Miss Mendoza, are you coming back after summer vacation?"

AJ, my Chuukese student asks me anxiously. Chuuk is an island in Micronesian and along with the Marshall Islands, Pohnpei, and Kosrae, make up at least half of my class. The boys are sometimes huge, and draw intricate tattoos on their bodies with indelible ink and scowl at me when I reprimand them. I worried they would get blood poisoning if they continued. I couldn't understand why they couldn't stop drawing or singing in class until I learned that in the Pacific, tattoos are an integral part of the culture; an art form that combines history and spirituality and that in cultures without

written languages, tattoos are a badge you wear to tell your story.
Other students are from Vietnam, Thailand, Japan, China, Taiwan, Cambodia, Macao, and The Philippines. It is a miniature United Nations and I am the mistress of ceremonies, performer, and mother in addition to my job as teacher.

Today my class is annoying, loud and needy. The 6th graders need hugs, the 7th graders need a good kick in their collective asses for rudeness and the 8th graders are perfect today because I bribed them with candy. We are working on an essay contest, and I am helping them to express themselves with words. The topic is, "What habit do you have that is unusual," and one bright Chinese girl Ophelia, (Many Chinese students give themselves a nickname) writes that she talks to herself, a boy says he is never hurt when someone is beating him up, that he doesn't feel pain and another says he is depressed because he hasn't any friends here that speak his language. One speaks of being too short, parents that are too strict, or never home because they are always working. I can't help them all but I catch what others sometimes don't: the signs of mental illness. I listen and when I have to, I act. When I can't, I give them acknowledgment and a voice. This takes me out of my head and illness. Hope, courage and sanity are the gifts that are in the hopeful eyes of my students.

One controversial tool I use is medication. A big debate in the mental health community is if psychotropic meds are necessary. I tried to heal without any and discovered that all my tools worked only so much without medication. I still had panic attacks. Now, I see a psychiatrist once a month and for the past ten years I found two medications that work. Why is it acceptable for a diabetic to take insulin, but if a person with a mental illness takes a drug, they are often criticized. I take ten mg of Lexapro and one mg of Clonazepan and I haven't had a full blown panic attack for seven years. I need medication and meditation. Both are vital to my mental and physical health.

My medication does not affect my personality. It just keeps me on the ground floor of life instead of the basement where my mind had once resided... I don't want to live in the basement anymore. I am still that girl; a hopeless romantic, but I'm not helpless or reckless anymore. I now have an inner spiritual guide who is wise and fearless. When I faced the truth I started remembering the good chapters in my past as well as the trauma.

Every summer, my mother made a birthday party for me. She had never had one and that was one thing she wanted me to experience; cake or no cake. My few school friends did not keep in touch during the hot summers.

So, my mother would go out and recruit strange kids to come to my party. "Come, you want candy, my daughter's birthday is today," and she would return with a scraggly bunch of hungry kids from the project. They were never the same kids as they year before and when they sang Happy Birthday they always stumbled on my name, but it was fun to be a stranger at your own birthday. As much as she harmed me, she helped me to buy my first and only house, as much as she rejected my desire to sing and dance, she rented the community center and bought candy to give me an audience. She was never predictable, but she was the best mother she could be. I doubted her love during the name calling, but I didn't know what mental illness was then either. She only said she was sick and only when I experienced first hand, the suffering that accompanies mental illness did I know there is no way to describe that kind of pain.

Telling the truth helped me appreciate the good that she did for me. My love of reading was something that she gifted me with, and I passed that legacy along to my own children and now to my students. There are many days, I dread leaving my cocoon, many days I question my recovery, many days I still feel anxious and depressed, but I am grateful and most of the time filled with awe at what I have accomplished since the Millennium.

In these ten years I have become self supporting for the first time, lived and worked in another country, lost sixty five pounds and found the spirituality and self respect I have been searching for my whole life.

Helping others helps, but self- love is mandatory. I am kind to myself first so I can be kind to others, and if someone remarks, “Another massage and dance class?” I say yes, and more.

I always knew what was bad for me, but now I don’t go there. Hate is not eating me up anymore. I have always been a searcher, but wasn’t able to tap into it because the lies contributed to my mental illness.

I used to hug trees in the projects, so amazed by the beauty of nature. In the sixties when hippies were into hugging trees, I didn’t want to because I was into the fantasy of finding, keeping and hugging the perfect man.

Zen means to be fully aware, to live in the present moment. It’s a process, a journey, not a destination. When I was stuck in the house engulfed by my anxiety, I was living in the future, thinking of what catastrophic event would happen to me next, and it usually did. When I was depressed I was stuck in the mysterious past, but by discovering my past, I was able to fight my mental illness. I was always walking around confused at the direction my anxiety disorder was taking me; my sadness so magnified, I couldn’t explain it to anyone. I think of all the tears, heartbreak and sleepless nights I blamed on a man's infidelities. I was told I was a drama queen, a crybaby, a lunatic.

Now, I understand my obsession with food and men were smokescreens to soothe and block out my chaotic, abusive childhood and the anxiety and agoraphobia that were produced from it. I sometimes lose the continuous fight to leave my house, but I let go of the guilt and self-hatred that laid the foundation for my illness.

I understand how genetics as well as trauma contributed to my mental illness and it helps to know it's not my fault, just as it wasn't my mother's fault. We were hostages to a powerful misunderstood disease. I survived, she didn't. I'm ok with the possibility that if no cure exists for me, I can still live a satisfying life keeping clear of closets.

I once lost my sight for a week because of trauma. I lost my voice because my mother spoke for me. I became bewitched by her words because even words that are untrue are powerful. I couldn't heal until I found my own words and my own truth. I lost my ability to breathe when I allowed men to define and abuse me and I abused myself with food to punish myself for my sins. I communed with boxes in my closet to save my sanity.

So, I went on a journey, to find the truth, wrote it down to understand it and remember. Now I know my sanity is connected to my truth. My truth is connected to forgiveness and forgiveness to love.

I no longer need the boxes I hid in to protect me from life. The protection was always inside of me; the divine essence, the core that kept me whole.

I won't let the stigma of mental illness define me. I will fight against that stigma. I can breathe, I am worthy and I am free...

I am walking to my favorite Pancake house "Boots and Kimo's." I'm sleeping over at my best friend Doni's house in Waimanalo, the wet, windward side of Oahu. On the way I stop by a bush of awapuhi blossoms and

think of a line of a standard Hula song, "Oh where are you beloved ginger blossom in the misty rain?"
I notice an old Hawaiian man looking at me.
"Sista, I no see many wahines' like you, really takin time for appreciating the aina (the land)." With my big smiling face I nod toward him.
This is my truth; my sanity. I tell it, I shout it; I own it. This is my Zen.

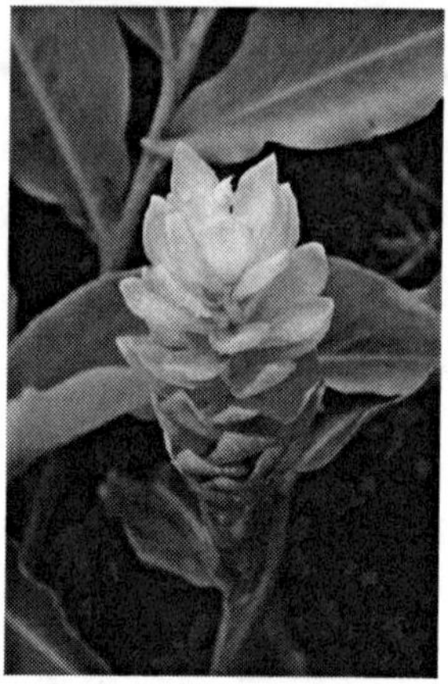

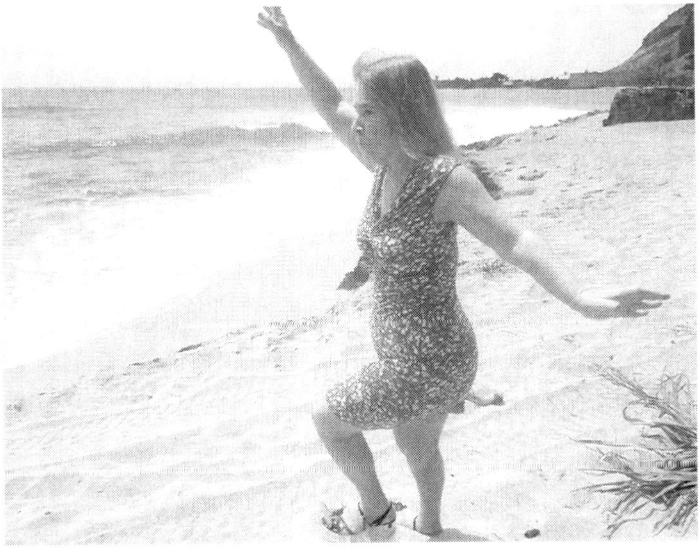

Epilogue

That was where my mother's diary ended. She entered the city hospital she feared a few days later. One day, my father went to visit her and asked the receptionist for Mendoza and he was given a different room number. My brother Angel or Angie as we called him was in that room next door to my mother's and had been there since the day he left. He died from peritonitis from alcoholism the day I arrived from Hawaii. My father said that if my mother hadn't been admitted that very day to that very hospital, we never would have found Angie. They say there are no coincidences.
My mother died three weeks after I arrived. Sometimes I wake up and hear her voice.
"Your face is so oily, you can cut the grease with a knife," and I automatically reach for the acne scrub, remembering I once wished for a real knife to cut my face off with. My therapist says these are the tapes that I carry around with me like a broken suitcase and I need to make other vacation plans.
I never knew the woman who wrote that diary. She kept a lot of secrets to protect me from the monsters who attacked her soul and I reciprocated by keeping my demons away from her.

Yet, she was more than her illness. She was witty, bright and funny. She taught me that reading can help you escape your illness for awhile, and that gift gave me the knowledge to change my life.

I used to wish I were a princess living in some far away land. Now, I carry around a ferocious hunger, not for food or men; but reality and life, an exquisite need to make up for my lost years in the closet.
And, I trust myself more and more to make the right decisions. When I found the love of my life; me, I was

ready for the love of the decent, kind man who is now in my life. Do I still dance in front of dark televisions? Yes, but with joy. And do I still crave French toast? Hell yea!

"Marilyn Mendoza's memoir is a beautifully written saga of one person's perseverance to victory over physical and mental illness. I have read dozens of memoirs, and this is one of the most inspiring. As you turn the pages you can't wait to see how she can possibly survive, but she does and writes to tell about it. A fascinating read."

Boyd Lemon
Author of critically acclaimed new memoir - Digging Deep: A Writer Uncovers his Marriages

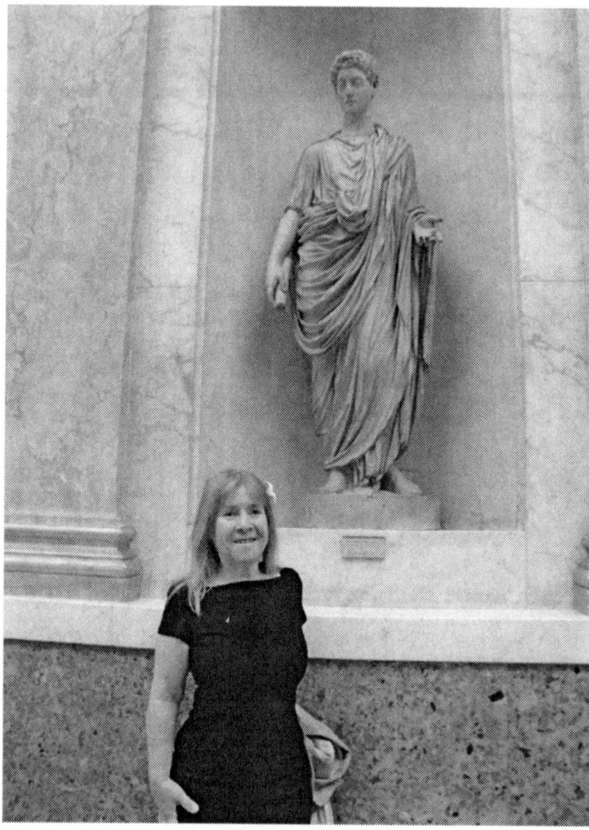

2010 Paris